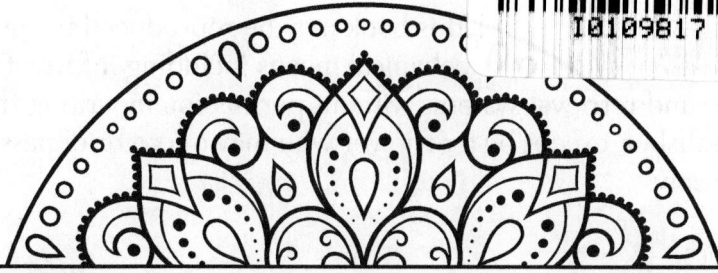

Yoga Beyond Body & Mind

The Yoga of Knowledge as Taught by Ramana Maharshi and its Relevance Today

by David Frawley
Acharya Vamadeva Shastri

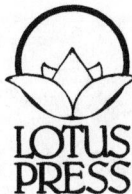

LOTUS
PRESS

© 2024

First Edition: 2025

ISBN: 978-1-6086-9255-2
Library of Congress Control Number: 2024946491

Cover design courtesy of Shankari Van Acker

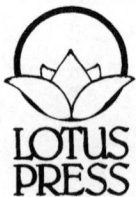

Published by:
Lotus Press
P.O. Box 325
Twin Lakes, WI 53181
www.lotuspress.com | lotuspress@lotuspress.com
Ph: (262) 889-8561

To Bhagavan Ramana Maharshi, the supreme sage of
Nondualist Vedanta and the highest Self-Realization,
and to Kavyakantha Ganapati Muni, the great master
of Mantra and all the secrets of Yoga, whose teachings
have guided me and inspired this book.

And to all the great Rishis, Yogis, Gurus, Seers and
Sages from the ancient Vedas to today, who guide
humanity beyond the darkness of ignorance, death,
duality and sorrow to immortality. May we follow with
unfathomable wisdom with complete dedication!

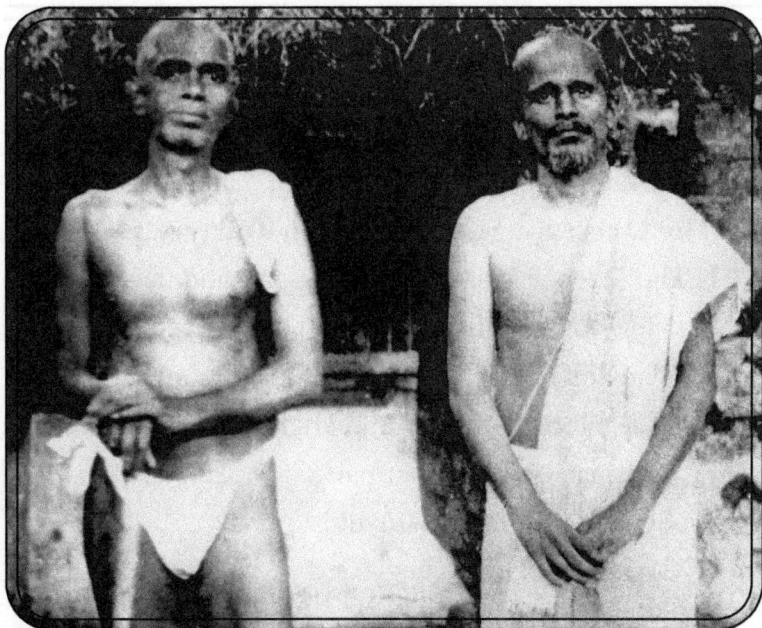

Ramana Maharshi and Kavyakantha Ganapati

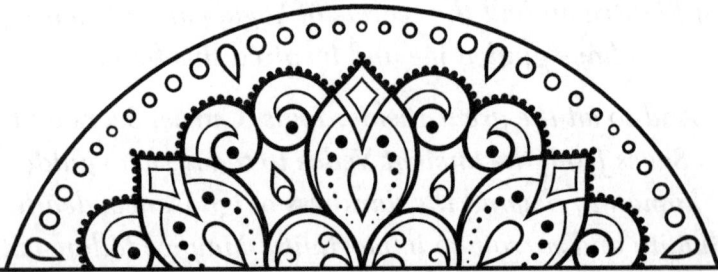

TABLE OF CONTENTS

AUTHOR'S PREFACE

Our aim is to explain the path of Self-realization in the tradition of *Advaita* (Non-dualist) Vedanta and the Yoga of Knowledge (Jnana Yoga), yet to do so in a way that is relevant and understandable today.

The book follows the traditional teachings of the *Upanishads*, *Bhagavad Gita* and *Yoga Sutras* in ancient times to the teachings of Shankaracharya (Adi Shankara) that set forth in detail and depth this Yoga of Knowledge. With these as a foundation, it emphasizes the Advaitic teachings as clearly explained in the teachings of Bhagavan Ramana Maharshi in the twentieth century, as the most recognized and honored modern guru of Self-realization. I have shared these profound teachings of Self-realization of Ramana Maharshi, who represents the Vedic tradition of non-duality and direct Self-realization in his life and teaching.

I have also tried to explain these transcendent teachings relative to our very different language, culture, and mindset today, which is engrossed in the material world, outer compulsions, and media images, far from any unity consciousness or non-duality. Yet there remains individuals and groups who are open to such higher teachings from Yoga and meditation backgrounds, and those looking for a universal consciousness.

First Part of the Book

The first part of the book consists of my study of Self-Realization relative to the teachings of Ramana Maharshi and *Advaita Vedanta* in the context of those seeking such Self-realization today, for whom it is something new, unusual, and hard to experientially grasp as it is beyond body and mind.

For people today in our very different information technology era we hope this first section of the book can form a bridge to these profound non-dualist teachings that look to a reality beyond all time, place, and person, which transcends our current world view and social order, including what we regard as our bodily or mental identity.

To create a bridge to that, I have provided an introduction and background to this transcendent knowledge in the first part of the book. This is to set forth the context, way of life, and support practices necessary to understand these teachings that have a very different view of the human being and the universe.

Second Part of the Book

The second part of the book consists of my translation and commentary on *Upadesha Saram*, the "Essence of Instruction", one of the most important works of *Ramana Maharshi*, which in less than forty verses explains the path of Self-realization according to Yoga and Vedanta. It shows the inner meaning and relevance of these profound teachings and helps us understand their very different language and terminology.

Such advanced Yoga of knowledge teachings were originally presented to Ramana's advanced disciples, who had many years of meditation and sadhana behind them. That is why the First Part of the book is helpful, if not necessary, to approach these.

Author's Views

My views in this book are meant to stimulate deeper introspection and Self-inquiry on the part of the reader, not to impose a mere set of ideas or concepts for intellectual scrutiny. There is no ideological or doctrinal debate included in this study. The focus is on the inner practice, the "sadhana of Self-realization," through the process of Self-inquiry.

The author does not claim to represent Ramana Maharshi or his teaching in any formal manner, though I have been connected to teachers in his lineage over the last fifty years. Such supreme teachings are beyond any personal appropriation and belong to the realm of Eternity.

The importance of Self-realization is for you the reader in your own deepest awareness and core life-experience, to help you see beyond our transient, uncertain, and dualistic material world shadowed in spiritual ignorance. This helps you to reclaim your true nature as Pure Consciousness, the boundless light of Self-awareness one with all.

Self-inquiry, the search for our true immortal Self, is an inner process, not a mere mental process, as the mind is shadowed by ignorance and duality. It requires that we turn the mind within, which is essentially to offer the mind and its activities to the silent awareness within.

How to Understand Vedantic Teachings

Vedantic teachings are about the Self of all beings and all existence, the inner awareness at the core of all existence manifest and unmanifest, not our ordinary personal or collective identity or mindset. Yet relating to the inner Self varies according to the time, place, person, mind, and the language in which its reality is shadowed. The way to the Self begins with the mind, but requires setting the mind aside as something apart from you in order to reach the goal.

Clarity of examination and precision of meaning rare essential for this teaching to be understood at an experiential level. It is not an emotional high or intellectual fascination but a return to the hidden depths of our inner being that reach to the Cosmic Mind and beyond it to the Supreme Self (Paramatman), the reality Absolute.

ACKNOWLEDGMENTS

I would like to specially thank Sri Ram Mohan of the Sri Ramanashram in India for his introductory foreword which provides an indepth perspective for approaching Ramana's teachings and the Yoga of Knowledge overall.

Most important was K. Natesan (1912-2009) was my main guide in approaching the Maharshi's teachings since I met him over thirty years ago, providing me with deep insights and his personal experience of Ramana. He also carried the profound mantric teachings of Kavyakantha Ganapati Muni, the great Yogi who was Ramana's chief disciple and shared these with me as well.

Sadguru Sivananda Murty (1928-2015) was another great inspiration. He held the deepest Self-knowledge and the ability to communicate it to people today, as well as understanding the Vedic and Yoga traditions overall.

Relative to Advaita Vedanta, Swami Dayananda Sarasvati of Arsha Vidya (1931-2015) was my main teacher in that profound tradition, with a discerning mind and depth of teachings.

Dr. David Frawley
(Acharya Vamadeva Shastri)

May 2024

FOREWORD BY DR. RAM MOHAN

This remarkable book "Yoga Beyond Body and Mind" takes the spiritual aspirant in a guided tour of the transcendental subject of the *Advaita Vedanta* view of Self-Realization. It is a profound presentation, explaining in lucid terms the fundamental concepts of *Sanatana Dharma,* such as *Jivatman* and *Paramatman,* 'sookshma shareera' (subtle body) and 'karana shareera' (causal body), the locus of the mind, stimulating the practitioner's enquiry through profound questions like "is our reality or identity physical?"

While the presentation is based upon the transcendental teaching of Yoga, Vedanta and the *Bhagavad Gita,* it is embellished with a detailed presentation of the spiritual teachings of the greatest *Advaitic* preceptor of modern times, Bhagavan Sri Ramana Maharshi. This book of Dr. David Frawley (Acharya Vamadeva Shastri) is an epitome of the non-dual teachings and direct path of Self-enquiry. It is presented in a ladder-like ascent from the fundamental to the Absolute, the vehicle being the teachings of Bhagavan contained in the thirty verses of *Upadesha Saram.*

The teaching culminates in the dissolution of the ephemeral ego in the Bliss Absolute. Dr. Frawley's book has logically developed into three sections: The first part deals with the author's perception of "Atmanubhava" or Self-Realization based on the ancient teachings of *Upanishads* and *Bhagavad Gita.* The second part delineates his profound analytical commentary on the succinct teaching of Bhagavan Ramana contained in *Upadesha Saram.* The author makes the imparting of this profound philosophy easily understandable through his lucid commentary.

The commentary on the *Upadesha Saram* deals first with the preparatory steps of explaining various aspects of Yoga like Karma Yoga, Bhakti Yoga, Mantra Yoga, Pranayama and Dhyana Yoga, leading the practitioner to the Direct Path of Self-Enquiry lucidly explained from Verse 17 onwards. The exposition of Self-enquiry in the verses of Upadesha Saram concludes with the remarkable statement "The Pure Awareness beyond the separate Self is the highest knowledge and deepest wisdom." Thus Dr. Frawley succeeds in presenting an entire vista of Vedantic Teachings contained in various spiritual texts in a nutshell with remarkable clarity.

I find Part 3, dealing with the important aspect of "how to apply the spiritual teaching to actual practice" a very important and a useful gift to the reader. A clear understanding of the ideas presented in the book constitutes a comprehensive understanding of the path to attain Self-Realization in a suitable manner consistent with the practitioner's level of awareness and way of living.

Dr. Frawley (Vamadeva) suggests three ways to do this while studying *Upadesha Saram*.

- Firstly: to absorb the essence of the whole text with total undivided attention and make it one's own spiritual guide.

- The second method, for those who are not so well advanced, is to concentrate upon one specific verse until "it permeates your awareness," followed by step-by-step focusing similarly on all thirty verses, thus in the process absorbing the 'Saram' or the essence of the entire text.

- The third method suggested by the author is to take a single verse and analyse the teaching according one's own level of awareness until it is completely absorbed, making the teaching and the teacher into one's own inner being. Dr. Frawley's commentary thus does the hand-holding from the initial preparatory steps of sadhana of the aspirant until the ultimate Self-Realization

I am reminded of the verse in Mooka Panchasathi of Mooka Kavi where the poet wonders at the Grace of Goddess Kamakshi who showed him the path to Self-Realisation through the Guru.

satkṛtadēśikacaraṇāḥ
sabījanirbījayōganiśśrēṇyā

apavargasaudhavalabhīmārōhantyamba
kē'pi tava kṛpayā || 97 ||

The poet says "Oh Divine Mother! those who have surrendered to the Guru receive your Grace. They are able to ascend the ladder of dual or non-dual sadhana, as per their qualification, and reach the pinnacle of Self-Realisation."

Dr. Frawley epitomizes the presentation of the Yoga of Self-Realization thus lucidly presenting the path to the discerning aspirant.

Starting with the fundamental description of "What is Self?" categorizing the mental, physiological or social self, he leads the practitioner by an evolutionary method to the Absolute. In a very compact manner this book clearly delineates various modes of looking into the term 'Self', the subtle body and Higher Self, related to the experiencing of one's Karmas. The important analysis of Jivatman, Paramatman and ego, the difference between individual consciousness and cosmic consciousness, the exploration into the 'Divine Within' - All these complex ideas are explained with great lucidity.

A very interesting portion of the book is the delineation of Transcendental Self-Realisation as in Yoga and Vedanta. It leads us to the understanding that there is a higher consciousness beyond our temporal life, beyond our mental constraints unto which we should all strives to reach.

Sri Ramana Maharshi's *Upadesha Saram* brings forth the fact that the spiritual hour for humanity's transformation has arrived. The resplendent verses of the epitomized Vedanta in *Upadesha Saram* are sounding forth the golden chines of the Eternal Spirit, calling to the all spiritually active and consecrated sadhakas.

This profound book of Dr. Frawley prompts the multitudes to listen to the Maharshi's call with confident and dynamic alertness. In these hours of the Earth's great crisis, threatened by a destructive global war, through discord and chaos, the call of the divine philosophy of Yoga and Vedanta as presented in the book facilitates an effectively encircling network of practical Vedanta to uplift humanity in the hour of crisis.

The presentation of a mystic mission advanced in this book to liberate humanity is echoed in the words of the poet William Blake:

"To open the eternal worlds, to open the immortal eye of man inward into the world's thoughts into Eternity. Ever expressing on the bosom of God, The human imagination."

This important book "Yoga Beyond Body and Mind" succeeds in expressing the inexpressible. To incorporate the lofty principles of the Vedanta, expressed by Bhagavan in just thirty couplets is no ordinary task. It is like draining the fathomless ocean into a dew drop. Not only that! Dr. Frawley also has mastered the art of presenting the prima-incomprehensible in a manner that renders it comprehensible even for a not yet discerning reader, through his concise, lucid and precise presentation.

There is no exhibitionist eloquence but a masterful presentation of the Master's Teaching. In a regulated flow of ideas, the book refines the secret of Karma, the pinnacle of Bhakti, the ultimate way of meditation and the summit of Self-Realization. Reflecting on the verses of *Upadesha Saram*, the author shows the reader the confluence of seemingly different practices in religion right from the (purva mimamsic) ritualistic, to the (uttara mimamsic) direction to the path of Self Enquiry.

The differences in the modes of the practice are based on the individual "adhikaras" or prerequisites. Nevertheless, all alight on the One and Only target of Self Realisation, the experience of unadulterated Cosmic Oneness.

Dr. Frawley (Acharya Vamadeva) concludes, in a sine-qua-non, "We require an inner guidance to move forward, a connection with an actual teacher who has either realised the Truth or represents a traditions or lineage holding the knowledge ("srotriyam brahmanistham" though not a necessarily in that order.). Bhagavan Ramana can lead us in this process, whether we look to him directly or to the teachers in his tradition, who can help us in our sadhana, extending to all ancient or modern Masters of Advaita Vedanta."

I recollect an analogy. In the Himalayas where flows the great holy rivers like Ma Ganga, it is not possible for everyone to get access to the ultimate sources of these divine rivers. Those who are fortunate and endowed with strength of body and mind reach these heights and bring the holy water down in barrels, which they fill into several small copper containers and distribute sanctified to all those living in the plains below. Likewise the great philosophy of Vedanta contained in the obscure time-defiant verses of the Vedas in Sanskrit can remind the uncomprehending majority if made accessible to them.

Teachers like Dr. Frawley take the effort to reach this world's majority to present the demystified Truth of the Vedas in a lucid way. Vamadeva through this book has accomplished a divinely empowered service.

Dr. Ram Mohan

Editor, "Ramanodayam" and Editorial Board
of "the Mountain Path". Director, Saraswati Research Centre.
Director, Centre for Study of Religion and Society.

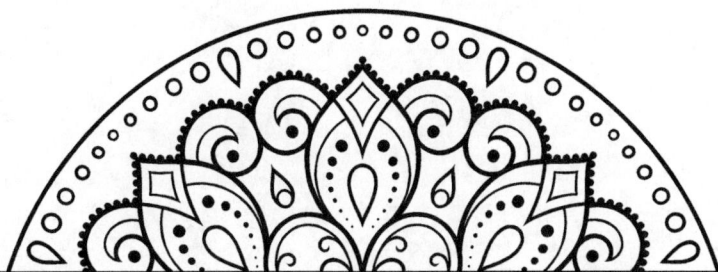

PART I
The Quest for Self-Realization Today

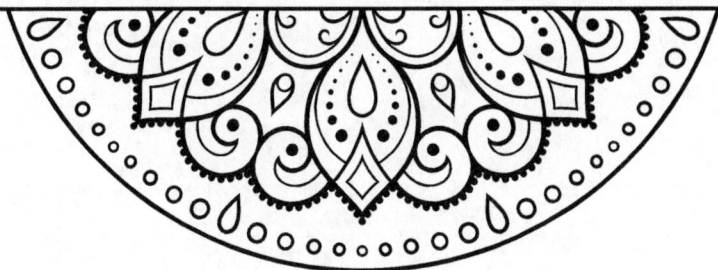

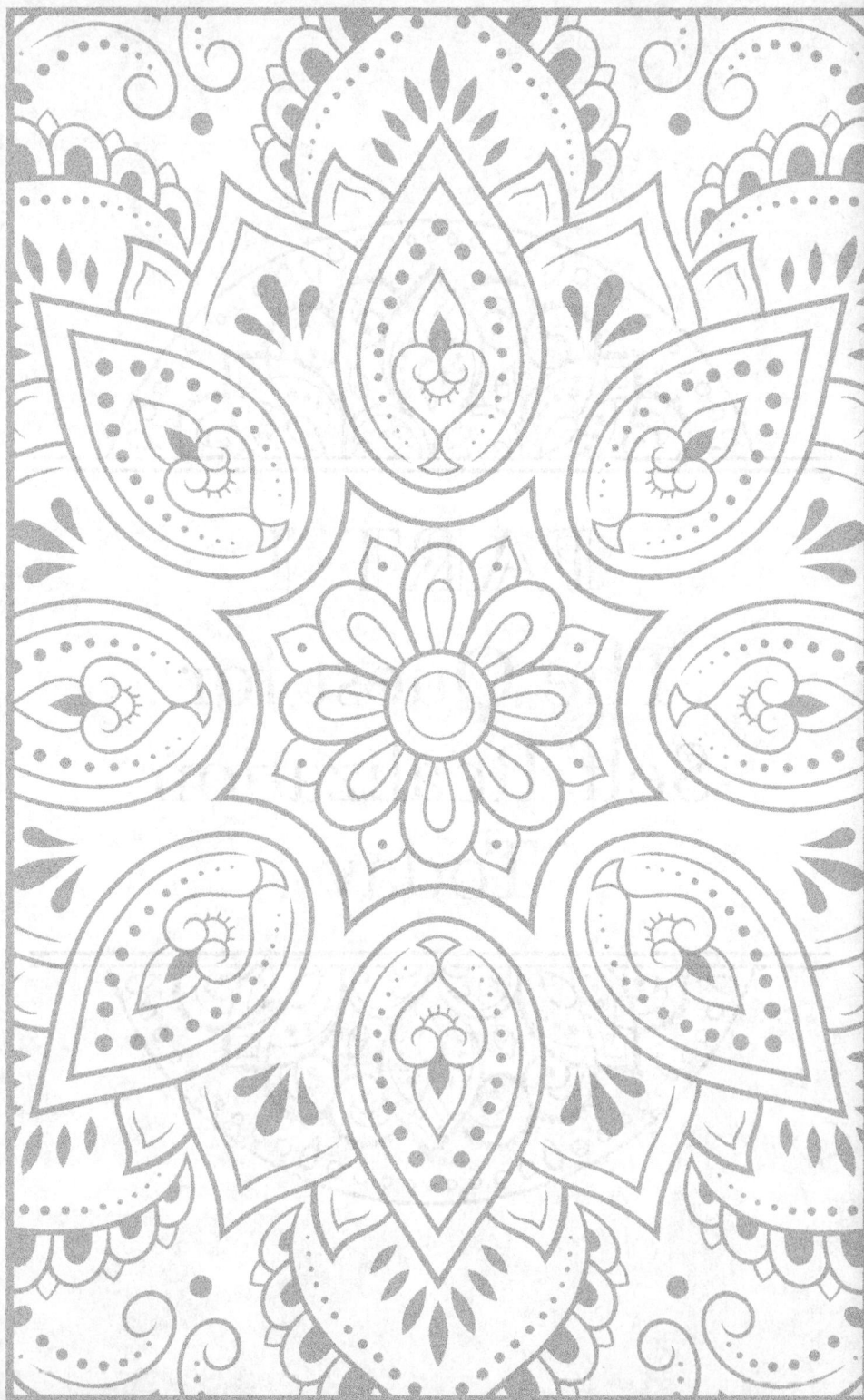

1.1

The Deeper Meaning of *Self-Realization*

Many people today teach what they may call self-realization, self-empowerment, or reaching your highest potential in life. While there are many interesting views and ideas in this regard, Self-realization in the higher sense of Yoga and Vedanta is usually more than these approaches and should not be reduced to them, however much value this new movement of self-examination and self-awareness may be in encouraging to look within.

The term Self for the *Atman*, the eternal and infinite Self-awareness behind the entire universe, is not easy to grasp, to even to conceive of in its true scope. This difficulty is based upon several factors, starting with how the term "self" is used in English and other modern languages, and amplified by the context of our modern media civilization that is dominated by an outward vision of the human being and self as a social projection or physical appearance.

While the Atman completely transcends what is called the ego in our current linguistic parlance and in our system of education overall, ego and self are usually regarded as the same, an equation that is seldom questioned. We do not use the term self as Atman in the transcendent sense of the Yogic and Vedic teachings. Quite the contrary, for us the self is first of all the personal self, mainly the bodily self, its related mental or psychological self, and our social self or social identity, which are all linked together.

Most of what we do and think about in life is based upon the pursuit of the self-interest of this personal bodily self whose reality we seldom question. This personal self constitutes the foundation of our ordinary existence. It is what society and other people consider to be who we are, emphasizing our role in the outer world of human interactions, not an inner reality in consciousness.

The term "self-empowerment" today usually refers to empowering this personal self aiming at success and achievement in the outer world through wealth, status, or social recognition. These constitute the main goals of our human life and striving. Our minds remain fixated on the external world as the true reality, however transient it may be, forgetting the fact of our own mortality.

Today self-realization usually refers to realizing the potential of our personal self in terms of our career, vocation, creative or mental skills. While there is nothing wrong with this view relative to the necessities and capacities of our outer lives, where it can be crucial and necessary, it orients our awareness in a very different direction than the search for Self-realization as the Atman or Self of all as in Yoga/Vedanta. Some groups that promote self-fulfillment or self-empowerment may refer to self-realization as something spiritual, but seldom with clarity as to what condition or fulfillment this realization is about.

Views of a Higher Self, Soul, or Spirit

Some groups use the term "higher Self" for a deeper spiritual nature beyond the personal and social self. Yet there is rarely depth or precision as to what this higher Self is, and how it relates to the universe as a whole. But such terms as higher Self do indicate an innate sense of a higher being or reality within us beyond our transient physical lives and social interactions. It reflects a deeper yearning for Self-realization in the universal sense, the quest for immortality and unity with all.

Many religions recognize a soul or spirit that endures beyond our physical life and has a continued existence after death, extending to heavenly realms. Such heavenly abodes, however, are not Self-realization in a yogic sense, but a reward for adopting and following a particular belief or faith. These can be subtle illusions, fantasies of the mind, or wishful thinking, and do not require any serious self-examination or questioning of our personal identity.

Such after death realms may portray a continuity of the physical personality or even physical body after death, rather than a higher Self as an inner being beyond name and form, body and mind, or any type of world-based embodied creature. These heavenly worlds are usually connected to the idea of only one life for the soul or inner being, and no concept of karma or rebirth.

There are views of the soul of a person surviving after death in some form or another from ghosts to angels, but still very far from the Self of Vedanta which is beyond any limited identity. Such views suggest another reality beyond our human lives, but do not recognize our eternal essence of pure Self-awareness. They can still reflect an ego consciousness.

In this regard, we must also acknowledge traditional and indigenous cultures throughout the world, who connect the spirit in human beings with various deities, nature spirits, sacred ancestors, or sacred powers of nature, which form an integral part of their lives, behavior, cultures, and view of the universe.

While the Atman is more than a nature spirit or even the manifest universe in all its beauty and wonder, such intuitions of consciousness hidden in nature reflect the deeper truth that our identity is not limited to the physical body or individual person, and has a connection with the whole of life, a true inner nature one with the cosmic nature. Whenever we approach nature with an open mind and heart, concentrating holding our awareness there, as native people do, we can sense that Supreme Self behind all even if we do not have a clear understanding or recognition of it.

The Atman is the ultimate essence behind nature and the cosmos, beyond any limited time, location, and person. This inner Self is often compared to a force of nature like light, space, energy, lightning, or vibration, more so than anything that can be described in human terms, more a universal force, presence, and guiding intelligence than a particular human form or function of the human mind.

Artists often possess an inspirational sense of oneness with nature, particularly painters and their landscapes. They have an intuition that our bodily identity is only a point focus of a great universal identity expanding far into time and space, extending perhaps to the whole of nature or beyond. They may identify such beauty and vastness as the truth of art. But while they can represent this sacred vision of nature in their artwork, they rarely realize it inside themselves or enter into a higher Self-awareness as their daily reality.

One could say they can see the cosmic reality through a window but cannot enter into it. This is because realization of that Self behind nature requires deep meditation. While it is not difficult to touch upon it, it is very difficult to hold it in a moment-by-moment awareness.

The Self and Dharmic Traditions

Many spiritual groups, particularly in Asia, accept rebirth or reincarnation, connected to the law of karma. Karma is the key term in the dharmic traditions from India as the Hindu, Buddhist, Jain, and Sikh, which discuss different types of karma and rebirth in great depth. They do not see the following the laws of some deity in the distance as the measure of right behavior, but rather a respect for all living beings and the interdependence and unity of the whole of life.

While even dharmic traditions, like the Buddhist and Jain, may not accept the Atman or Self as specifically described in yogic and Vedic traditions, they do emphasize karma and rebirth as the basis of our existence, which is not limited to the physical body, and teach a path to transcend birth and death to an enduring consciousness, or enlightened state through meditation practices as taught by their great gurus, sometimes called our Self-nature as in Zen Buddhism.

Most of the differences between dharmic philosophies are semantic or philosophical, or alternative approaches. They all teach that there is a supreme state of truth or highest dharma beyond the mind, known only in the state of Samadhi in which the mind is put to rest and its karmas transcended.

Other groups accept that there is a reincarnating soul or inner being, continuing aspects of the physical personality into successive births. They may consider that such rebirths continue perpetually, without a clear view of any Self-realization beyond the separate individual being, or may have our rebirths end in a higher world or loka, much like a heavenly realm. They may be part of occult teachings about various mysteries of life and death. For them reincarnation may not need to be transcended but explored.

The Subtle Body and the Higher Self

Along with the idea of a reincarnation is that of a subtle body or other finer vestures of the soul or spirit beyond the physical – connected to energy, light, and intelligence. This idea of a subtle or energy body extends to subtle or astral worlds after death, realms of imagination like heavens or hells, which can also relate to experiencing the results of one's karmas there before returning to Earth to enter another physical life. It reflects the dream state in our personal lives and sleep as a world of experience. It reminds us of religious heavens and hells but with deeper implications.

Yoga proposes a causal or seed body or vesture beyond the subtle body as the ultimate repository of karmic patterns and the basis of rebirth. This causal body is usually viewed as consisting of a deeper intelligence, connected to realms of higher meditation and the original creative seed forces behind the universe. As it is formless, it is closer to the Vedic view of the Atman but is not beyond duality or individualized existence.

Such views take us in the direction of a higher Self and propose a more enduring identity for us beyond the physical self or mental self. In the Advaitic view, our true Self or Atman transcends all embodiments, physical, subtle, and causal.

Jivatman and *Paramatman*

Vedanta calls the reincarnating individual being as *Jivatman*, meaning the living Self. This is the Self identified with body and mind in different incarnations and in different subtle realms as well as the physical. The goal of Self-realization is to move from the Jivatman or individual Self to the Paramatman or Supreme Self beyond all embodiment, physical, subtle or causal, including beyond all karma and rebirth.

Yet the Jivatman is not simply the physical personality, ego or mind. The Jivatman is the individual consciousness that endures throughout the entire cycle of rebirth. To connect to the Jivatman, therefore, is already to reach an awareness far above our ordinary identification with the body and mind. It is to recognize that we have had many births, in many bodies and many worlds, and are not at all limited to this physical body or material world. It is to touch our immortality and ability to transcend death.

To recognize ourselves as the Jivatman is to awaken our aspiration to Paramatman and the pursuit of the Divine within, with Self-realization as our prime purpose and motivation in life. It connects us to our aspiration in every birth to ascend to a higher awareness and greater proximity to our transcendent Self. Once we recognize our identity as a Jivatman beyond the personal self of a single birth, the vistas of various yogic and spiritual practices open up for us in a practical manner, both to subtler realms and to the eternal and the infinite. Our life becomes a sadhana or yogic practice, not simply a seeking of outer enjoyments.

Yet to recognize our inner nature as Jivatman does not necessarily require that we remember the details of our previous human births, as these are transient physical factors, not part of our inner being. The physical mind and personality perishes along with the physical body, and has little relevance to future births that will follow their own karmas. The physical person is like a mask we wear for our physical life that we cannot carry with us to another incarnation.

To awaken at the level of the *Jivatman* requires that we remember core aspiration to realize the Supreme Self that is behind all our incarnations, what is called the meditation practice of "Self-remembrance". This also means being willing to forget the web of births that have kept us bound to our separate sense of self and the ignorance and sorrow that entails. It is an awakening at the level of the spiritual heart, not just a mental or emotional change.

Self-Realization in *Advaita Vedanta*

Ordinary views of self-realization relating to the fulfillment of personal self are not the Self-realization indicated in or sought after in Vedantic teachings. Such personal achievements are part of the not-Self or Anatman, the outer world of Maya, and very far from our true nature that is inherently beyond body and mind, birth or death. They pertain to the outer world not to our inner being. Vedantic Self-realization requires the negation and transcendence of the personal self, including its memories and karmas – a radical shift of identity from the transient to the eternal.

If you are truly in search of Self-realization in this Vedantic sense, you must let go of your personal self of body and mind as your true identity, and develop a detachment from its fears and desires, motivations, and ideas, striving and efforts. In short, you must transcend the ego on every side and in all that you do and think. You must detach your awareness from the thought-based mind and die to the outer self in order to reach your true nature, though this is a process of many lifetimes.

Very few, one in many millions or more, can achieve Self-realization as single event as Ramana Maharshi did as a mere youth of sixteen years old. To truly approach Self-realization, we must dedicate our lives to its pursuit as our main activity and aspiration, which we will carry on into the next incarnation as needed.

Yet this does not mean to pursue Self-realization one must necessarily give up one's work or our duties, which we are karmically involved with, varying by individual, time, and place. It does not require that we cannot function as needed in the practical world. It means we should maintain a transcendent vision and higher goal within us, anchoring any karmically necessary outer activity within an inner awareness, not making the outer world our prime focus or dedication. Certainly, it requires that we simplify our lives, reduce unnecessary involvements, and personal desires. But we can integrate the search for Self-realization into our lives if we give it priority and do our outer work as a kind of Karma Yoga.

To reach the Supreme Self, we must look beyond the entire cycle of rebirth, including the religious view of heavens, or any world or loka, however subtle. We need to transcend name, form, action, time and space into an unbounded Self-awareness. We must move from the Jivatman to Paramatman. While this is a great challenge for which we must face many obstacles, it is our ultimate journey and adventure into the boundless that brings the supreme peace and contentment.

To properly understand the Vedantic view of Self-realization one needs a different sense of self, reality and consciousness than accepted in human society today, including in religious or scientific circles, and a steady orientation of the mind towards introversion, silence, and stillness. Yet to approach Self-realization in an authentic and enduring manner is a rare and great achievement for the individual human being, though it may still be far from the ultimate goal. Having such an aspiration is indeed a great blessing that will bear its fruit over time, and never be lost.

The purpose of this examination here is to instill that transcendent view of Self in the reader, removing the bondage to the lesser self and personal mindset. Otherwise, the profound and exalted teachings of Advaita can be easily misinterpreted or scaled down to a lesser sense of self, even if that sense of self is of subtle realms beyond our physical world. Do not demean or diminish the transcendent Self within you, by never turning within to acknowledge it. Its light will arise and illuminate your mind if you offer your life to it, or at least honor it above all.

Levels of the Universe

Vedantic texts, which form the foundation for students of Self-realization, explain the factors of our greater existence in detail. Below we summarize the main factors involved.

The Seven Levels of Existence:

1. Anna or matter and substance.
2. Prana or energy, vitality, and magnetic forces.
3. Manas or informational data and processes.
4. Vijnana or inner creative intelligence.
5. Ananda or bliss as all-pervasive.
6. Chit or pure consciousness beyond all form or objectivity.
7. Sat or eternal being, immutable, Absolute.

The Five Koshas or sheaths of the embodied self:

1. Annamaya kosha as the physical body sustained by food (food).
2. Pranamaya kosha as vital energy, sustained by the breath.
3. Manomaya kosha as outer mind and cognitive senses.
4. Vijnanamaya kosha as experiential intelligence.
5. Anandamaya kosha, essence of delight.

The Three Bodies or shariras:

1. Gross or physical body, mainly substance and food based but holding deeper energies and mental processes, waking state.

2. Subtle or astral body, mainly vital energy but also sensory and imaginative part of the mind, dream state.

3. Causal or formless, seed consciousness prior to name, form or energy, deep sleep state.

The process of karma and rebirth works through these different interrelated levels of existence, body mind. We need to purify the mind, surrender the ego, and become detached from not only the physical world but all potential worlds and lokas. Yet as subtle and causal realms are quite magical, radiant, and transformative, one can easily become in their processes, and remain there long after physical life has ended.

Prime Vedantic texts like the *Vivekachudamani* (Crest Jewel of Discrimination) of Shankaracharya can be examined for this in greater detail. It is crucial that we learn not just about the outer physical body and corresponding material world, which is only a small part of the reality of Brahman or the Absolute but recognize the greater existence that dwells within us to Pure Being itself that is the substratum of all and our true immortal Self.

We need to understand our inner journey through time and space, birth and death, and all realms of existence, as our inner being strives to unfoldment its transcendence state of Self-realization, not just relative to the physical or the human realm but to all manifestation and the unmanifest itself beyond the known.

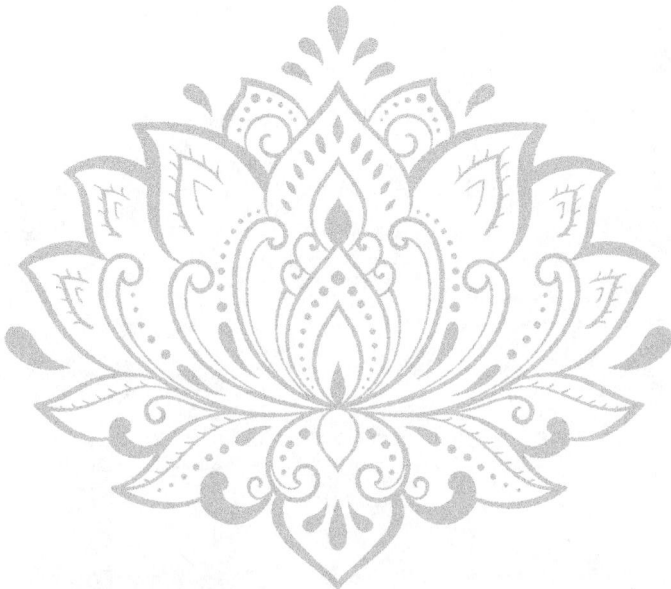

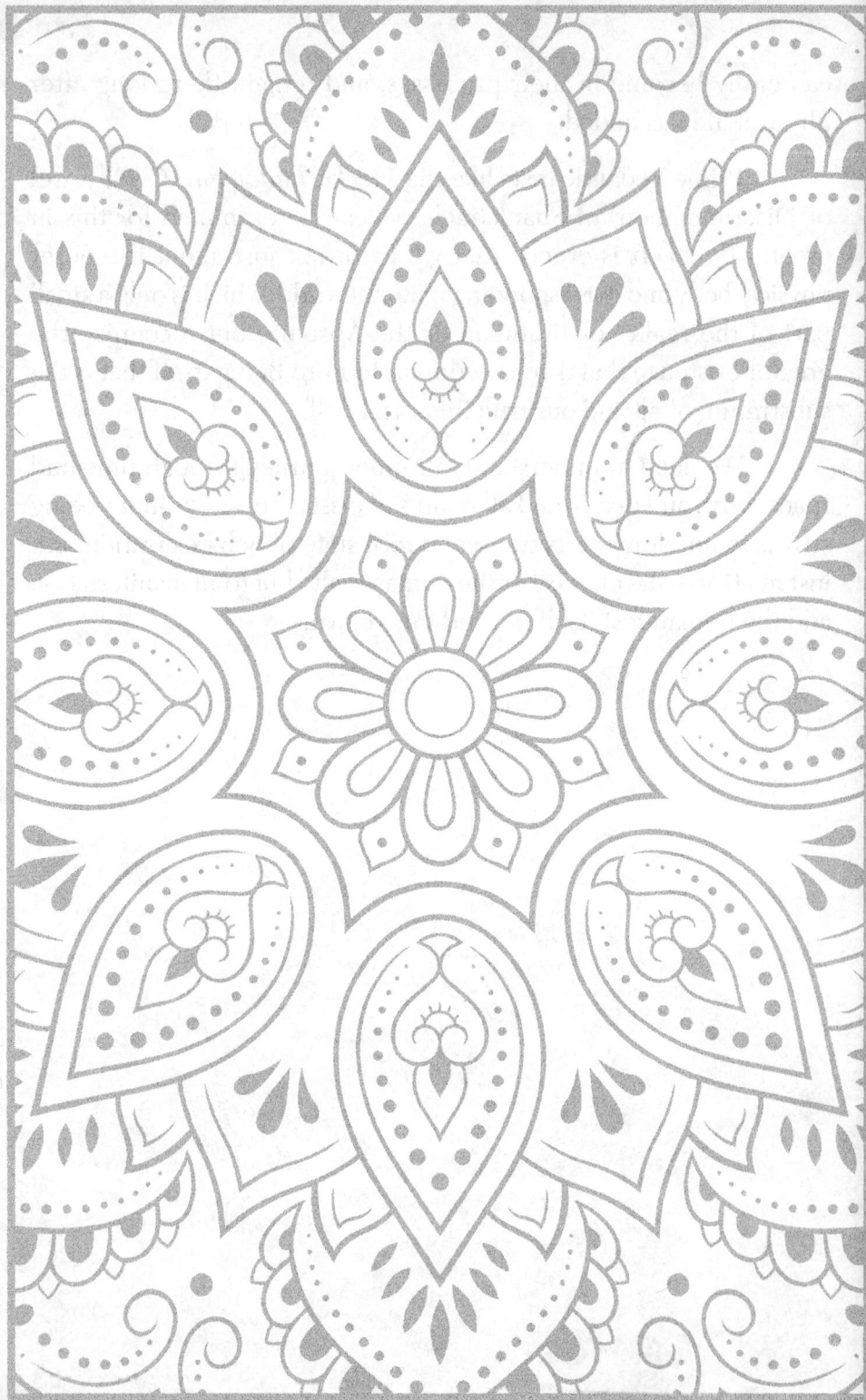

1.2

Beyond the Intellect to Pure Awareness

Modern civilization is based upon the intellect or rational mind as its primary means of truth discernment and verification, by which we can determine what is real or unreal, true or false, making it into the final arbitrator of the meaning of our lives. Through it we create various instruments, machines, categories, laws, and theories to explain how the world of nature works, and how to understand the workings of the human body and mind.

Culturally we regard the human intellect as our most important and accurate power of intelligence with its detailed ideas, theories, calculations, categories, and conclusions. Our highest human type is the intellectual genius like Albert Einstein, and we name great scientific discoveries after their research. What we call education is the development of this intellect, with language, logic, research, experimentation, and exploration.

The intellect is the basis of science and technology and all branches, which remains at the pinnacle of our view of what is true knowledge in this computer age. The intellect develops various equipment, mathematics, terminology, and systems of measurement, to verify objectively or outwardly the truths it proposes, taking us beyond the limitations and biases of the human mind and senses.

We employ the intellect to examine all domains of life, our behavior, progress, and evolution, as if it were the ultimate judge and gold standard that everything must be verified by. As such, the intellect is the basis of our modern scientific education, from which

15

we have removed religion and mysticism, and downplayed art and the humanities. It is the basis of our mass media, its images, conclusions and so-called facts that it pursues.

We strive to expand and verify the theories of the intellect by the instruments it has constructed, and their providing of evidence and proof. Yet intellectually defined evidence remains a work in progress and over time the great conclusions of intellectual knowledge of one era must be revised, transcended, or even rejected. Scientific experiments and even medical testing can give different results at different times and places or relative to different people, cultures, circumstances, and environments.

The question then arises, what is the true capacity of the intellect, its powers, and limitations? Is there any other form of intelligence we can access within us beyond the intellect. The intellect remains limited and personal in its basis and has its biases that can prevent us from understanding the whole or totality. The intellect is only a specialized instrument, not a direct means of knowing, perceiving, or experiencing the truth.

The intellect does not provide direct and indisputable knowledge, but only competing conceptions some which may be regarded as proven and many of which are not or are disproven in the course of time. The intellect has own truth verification system based upon its own instruments and measurements, making it into a self-regulating discipline. Its peer group studies may only reinforce the opinions or prejudices of the peer group. In short, the intellect is bound by its own inherent ego, preferences or biases that limit its scope of insight and realization in the yogic sense of consciousness is not even recognized in the modern intellectual world.

Intellectuals have their various arguments, opinions, and debates, which are seldom final and can be quite contentious. Most intellectuals are competing with or in conflict with other intellectuals and their different theories, opposing or trying to disprove them. Intellectuals can be jealous or angry. I sometimes say that intellectuals are the most emotional people, in spite of the idea that the intellect is detached from emotions. All you need to do is question or reject their pet theories or their academic or political correctness, and you will find the intellectual emotionally reactive and disturbed like everyone else.

As individuals in our intellectualized world today, we are rewarded for intellectual success and achievement. Intellectual knowledge or competence has its own financial, social, and even political power, which gives a person a reason to promote their intellectual views for personal advantageous. That is not to target intellectuals but simply to recognize human nature based upon the ego, which modern intellectuals seldom question or look for a truth beyond the ego.

The intellect is the rational and conceptual mind and thought process. That is perhaps the simplest way to look at it. It forms ideas and categories and recognizes names, forms and numbers and their combinations. The modern intellect is essentially an intelligence of the human brain, and is affected by its physical, emotion and social influences, though intellect as such has connections beyond the brain that we do not understand.

The ability to influence the intellect through experimenting with the brain, using brain altering or regulating drugs and medications is a result of this intellect and brain equation. Yet its dangers are also well known. We can control the brain and related intellectual knowledge and opinions chemically or medically.

In addition, we have now developed computers and artificial intelligence (AI) to expand, verify or transcend the intellect. The intellect can now be enhanced or controlled by its own mechanical creations that afford it greater powers of calculation. These may be free of certain personal or emotional prejudices, but may also create an inhumane, non-feeling type of intelligence that places outer organization over the human rights of any person. Some countries like the United States have already given corporations the rights of a person, which we may eventually do so with certain computer-based creations, giving them a power of decision over us that can be dangerous.

Intellectual Knowledge, Its Nature and Limitation

What exactly is it that we can claim to know through the human intellect? While intellectual knowledge can be very complex, it can also be seen as a type of intellectual reductionism. Intellectual knowledge is mainly information or data about the outer world and our outer physical and social selves. It is data, not necessarily understanding or respect for life and the individual. Such data includes all the domains of science such as physics, chemistry, geology, biology, medicine, and psychology, which are getting progressively more mechanical in this information technology era that the intellect has produced. The real person or immortal Self is not and cannot be counted, because it is the seer, not the seen.

Intellectual knowledge also includes philosophy as understanding the nature of reality, including ontology or knowledge of being, and considering how to access it through the intellect. But such qualitative applications of the intellect have been reduced by the quantitative orientation of the intellect in modern science in and imitation of technology, as we human beings were just machines and knowledge about us is only data, not anything creative or transcendent.

The outward-looking intellect has developed a vast technological world order through its ability to uncover the subtle energies of nature, like electricity or nuclear power, and access these through various machines and instruments, mechanical in nature. These new forms of equipment are devised by the intellect to expand its knowledge and power and even weapons productions which continue to grow rapidly today. The computer and cell phone are manifestations of intellectual research, if not genius and aid in calculation and communication. But their ethical application cannot be controlled by the intellect or even respected by it. The intellect can produce nefarious new weapons as well.

In addition, with all our new intellectual knowledge and technological wonders, most of us are still dissatisfied about what we know and are suspicious if it is a fabrication or manipulation, perhaps even a type of mind control. We are certainly justified in questioning our quantitative and mechanical world order ruled more by machines and equipment than by real people or anyone we know.

We all wonder if there is something more to magic of life and all the diversity of nature, than intellectual concepts and calculations. Clearly nature is more than what the intellect can measure in any final way. Art as spontaneous creativity is more than a formula the rational mind and adds inspiration to our lives that cannot be quantified or made into an algorithm. Whether there is something Divine, Eternal, Infinite, or any universal Intelligence, Consciousness or Cosmic Mind has yet to be determined by the intellectuals of today, though it has long been raised as an idea or ideal, if not an article of faith, and has been the basis of the spiritual and yogic discipline of the intellect extending back over thousands of years.

Intellectual knowledge often seems abstract, dry, and lacking in feeling, more like a machine than a living being or person. It seems to be missing the deeper meaning, value and purpose or life, which is not just about information but wisdom and higher awareness. We have a deeper aspiration to something eternal and infinite, an absolute truth, that the intellect can only provide an intimation for us through its cosmological theories and speculations. This requires not merely a sharp intellect or intellectual devices like computers, but an inner seeing, direct knowing or what is called realization, starting with who we really are behind and beyond mind and intellect.

The Knowledge of Great Rishis and Yogis

Great yogis, rishis, seers, sages, and mystics worldwide over the millennia have taught us another way of knowledge and perception than the intellect. They show to create a transformation as to how the intellect works, to turn the intellect around from the outer world and orient it within so that it can access the infinite and eternal within our deeper awareness. This is an awakening of an inner intelligence beyond body and mind.

The basis for this reorientation of the intellect is the practice of meditation through asking fundamental and existential questions, like "Who am I?", "What within me if anything endures after death? What exists in the space between our thoughts or whenever mind and intellect are in abeyance as in sleep"? "Who or what is the knower behind our thoughts"?

The examination of such profound questions forms the prime teachings of Vedanta, such as modern gurus like Bhagavan Ramana Maharshi back to Adi Shankara and the Upanishads. Recent Advaitic gurus from India like Swami Chinmayananda and Swami Dayananda (Arsha Vidya).

To use the intellect to access higher reality, requires practicing deep introspection, including to question the validity, necessity or finality of our thoughts and emotions, where have they come from, what value they have, and how we can go beyond their limitations to a direct awareness.

Inquiry based meditation is one of the most important paths of Yoga, Jnana Yoga, the Yoga of knowledge. It requires a reorientation of the intellect beyond name, form, number, and speculation to merging into pure consciousness, and direct awareness.

If we look deeply into our true nature, we will discover that we are of the nature of the pure light and energy of awareness, beyond body and mind, time and space, which abides steady and immutable behind all the movements and changes body, mind, and the external world. This is the Vedantic way of Self-realization, silencing the mind and going beyond the intellect to unity consciousness.

However, as we study such Self-realization based teachings we must do so as part of a meditation practice. Mere academics do examine such yogic texts from a place of practice. They are more concerned about whether the author of the text was an historical person, where or when he lived, if he composed the entire text or part of it, if he borrowed his ideas elsewhere, if the text was altered over time and how it compares with the ideas of other thinkers east and west.

While these are all interesting considerations, they do not address the actual topic of the teaching at an experimental level, which is Self-realization through meditation and Samadhi. Academia seldom questions the mind and remains the proponent of the supremacy of the outward looking intellect, not researching higher states of consciousness at an experiential level.

Unless we learn to turn the intellect inward beyond name, form and number, we cannot understand non-dual Self-realizations traditions, which remain a foreign land to us that we are examining in the distant with a distorted vision. We must honor the great gurus of Self-realization ancient and modern from the Vedic Rishis to Bhagavan Ramana Maharshi. It is not enough to follow modern psychology, philosophy, or science as these do not recognize any universal conscious, much less know how to realize it.

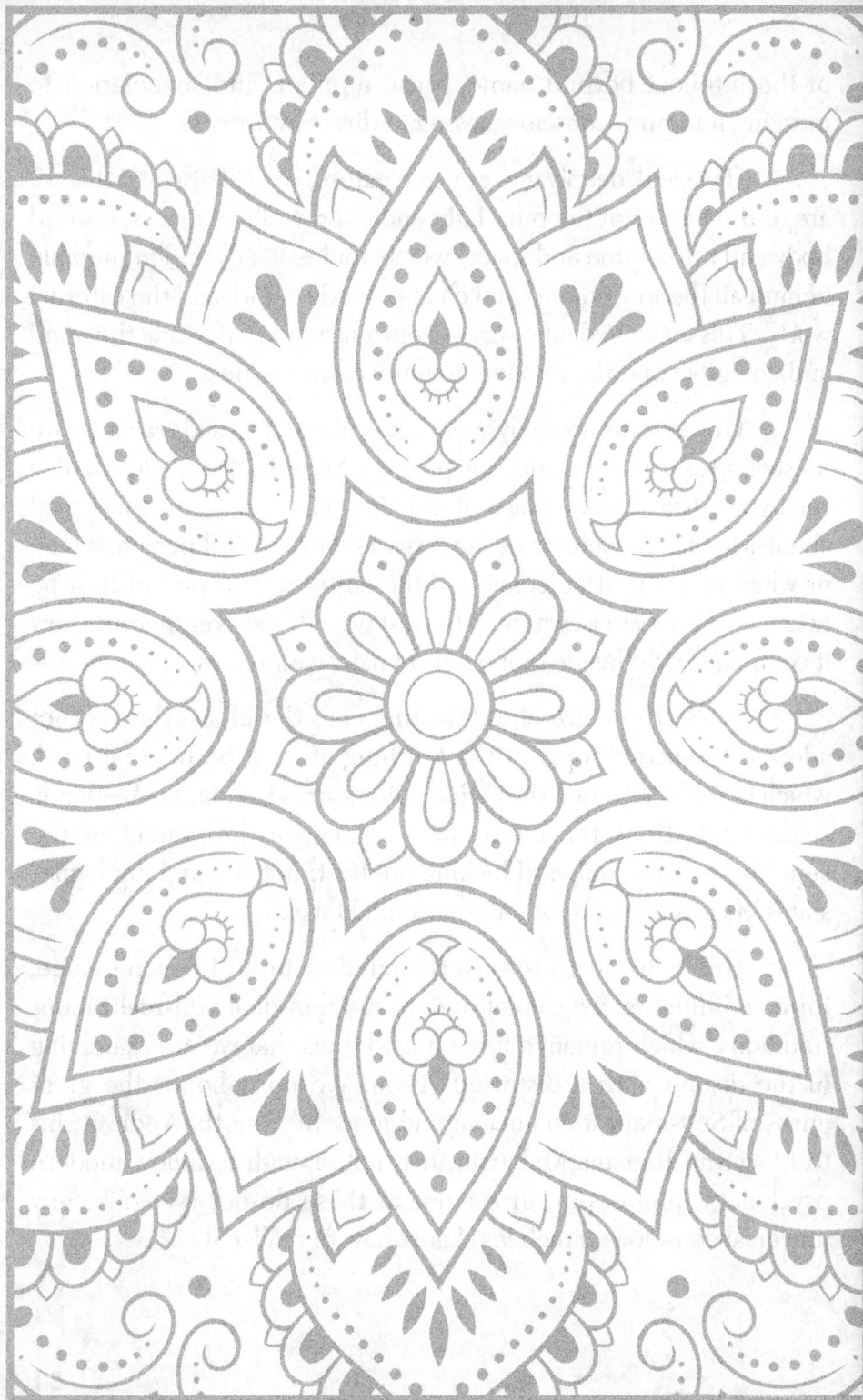

1.3
Is Our Reality Physical?

We are aware of ourselves as physical beings, centered in a physical body that has a precise and limited location in time and space. Our physical body undergoes various biological processes which shape our life experience. Our physical urges dominate us from birth to death in terms of our health, vitality, and ability to function in the outer world, which is a matter of survival. Our body has its unique genetic code governing its processes, which may predispose us to certain impairments or diseases.

Yet how we take care of the body in terms of diet, exercise and activity has a more important role as to how it functions. The questions arises then if we have to care for the body, we must be different from the body and not simply identifiable with it. Experientially, we are not just a body but a conscious being for which the body is an instrument.

The physical body is guided by a mind that is connected to the brain. This physical mind aims at protecting the body and fulfilling its biological urges, like hunger, thirst, and reproduction, without which we could not live in this material world. Yet in addition this bodily fixation is the foundation for the mind's mental functions, which can take us far beyond our mere physical concerns to probing into the greater universe in which we live, from the Earth to the distant skies beyond and a vaster reality than our mere mortal encasement.

We certainly must carefully take care of the physical body if we want to be healthy, happy and have a long life, even a clear state of mind. Our body requires the appropriate food, clothing, and shelter, including appropriate medicines to counter its disease tendencies and infirmities in the aging process.

The body is vulnerable to natural forces of heat and cold, wind and moisture as well as various diseases, chronic and acute, including numerous toxins and pathogens, which increase the longer we live. Our bodies need the right clothing for protection and can easily be injured or suffer accidents from outside forces, even if our internal physical health is otherwise strong. Protecting and preserving the physical body requires extensive ongoing efforts and occupies much of our time. Should we fail in this physical care, whatever else we may be attempting in life socially or mentally becomes compromised, ultimately causing the demise of our physical body bringing our physical existence to an abrupt end for something else we do not know. Our body consciousness is dominated by fears of what threatens it and desires for what gives it pleasure which control or minds and behavior.

Is Our Identity Physical?

Our bodily identity does not exist in itself and is not limited to our physical structure. We human beings are social creatures and depend upon the care or help of other people for our survival, growth and happiness. The individual physical being is not a self-sufficient entity but requires the support of other people to function.

Our social dependency begins with the family in which we are born, which raises us according to their capacities, inclinations, and resources, beginning with our parents who shape us at physical and psychological levels. Educating the human child can take twenty years or more for maturity and independence. Without extensive family care children cannot survive in their infancy or childhood. Our family forms the basis of our physical and social identity and its physical desires and necessities, though the family may have limitations of its own and may break down through divorce or disease, causing deep-seated traumas.

For the young human being to become independent or responsible requires a social-based education beyond the family in schools with classes with children of our same age and background. Our social interactions provide us our language and its meanings, teaches us how to speak, provides our values, and helps us develop an identity and place in the social order that defines us. This is not just a physical identity but a social identity that includes physical factors of age, place and time of birth and gender, but also our social status in terms of nationality, ethnicity, religion, education, financial state, skills and talents, level of intelligence and many other complex and changing social factors. These social factors are rooted in our physical identity but provide additional considerations that are not physical.

Society provides us a name, status, vocation, property, bank accounts, various types of identification, including social responsibilities to family, community and country. In other words, our physical identity extends at a social level to an extensive set of interactions and interrelationships with other people on various levels of responsibility that may put us under external influence or control, which may not be directly related to our physical or bodily condition.

This includes travel, moving our residence, or even a change of identity as when we relocate to another country, take on another job or assume another religious identity. Through our prime identity is physical, it is changeable over time and circumstances relative to our place in the world, and more of a practical necessity than an enduring inner reality. Our physical identity is part of an apparent self, a social projection, not an intrinsic self, and is fraught with assumptions and illusions at a social level, as well as ultimate disease and death at a physical level.

Location of our Minds

While our physical bodies have a single location in time and space that is clearly discernable, we also have minds that sustain a broader scope of action and awareness beyond our physical limitations. To begin with, we live more in our outward looking senses, than simply fixated on our own physical bodies. We are constantly adjusting and adapting to what the senses reveal and expose us to, which is constantly changing.

Our senses provide us a vast range of experience of a larger outer world beyond our personal control, which is diverse and engaging, and can be pleasurable or painful, even dangerous. We spend most of our time looking outward through our eyes and ears and evaluating our external environment, from the boundless world of nature to our strictly defined social and urban environments.

Part of this sensory engagement is simply to protect our physical needs, but it extends trying to understand the greater reality of life relative to which our physical presence is very small and precarious. We are but grains of dust in a vast unlimited universe and on a planet of billions of creatures. We can quickly become dispensable as greater social needs or compulsions arise, like soldiers on a battlefield.

We are usually only strongly focused on the body when we are engaged in specific physical actions or exertion, or when there is physical pleasure or pain. Otherwise, we happily forget our bodies and are caught up in our interactions with the outer world, now magnified by technology and the media. We are aware of ourselves not merely as a body among other bodies, but as one of a group or a community that we must support or even die for.

For us to be successful as physical beings, we must certainly be successful in the outer world. This includes in both human society and in our natural environment which have their differing opportunities and dangers. Therefore, we must be taught about the outer world and how it functions, from the setup of human society to the changes in nature according to the seasons or geographical locations, among many other factors of adaptation to the external forces that rule over us.

To properly use the senses and evaluate their inputs we have a mind that provides our ideas and experiences of self and world, which are interrelated. The mind allows us to coordinate our five senses and evaluate the data that comes through them, which is extensive, diverse and sometimes contradictory. We learn about the world and how its functions, including the laws of nature and the rules and regulations of society. We are taught in school such subjects as geography or history that take us beyond our present physical time and space locations, showing to us our actual small and temporary place in the world. The mind also allows us to imagine realms and experiences far beyond our physical capacities, whether cosmological or mystical.

Yet the mind not only engages the cognitive senses like the eyes and ears, it also directs and motivates our motor organs like the voice, hands and feet. The mind is not just an instrument of knowing but one of action. As such, the mind is colored by its own motivations, desires and expectations. Our actions in society can become more important than our own physical condition, notably our mental communication and expression can be more significant than our physical condition. Our desires color the mind and can cloud our sensory perception.

We have developed mechanical instruments that increase our sensory powers like telescopes and microscopes and every sort of vehicle for extending our motor organs or amplifying our power of speech. *Even the body serves as an instrument for the mind, its knowledge and actions, which brings into question our bodily identity. Are we the body or is the body an instrument of the mind? And is the mind perhaps the instrument of a higher consciousness?*

The Impact of Information Technology

Our society has changed significantly in recent centuries since the industrial revolution. It has progressively reduced our dependency upon physical labor and bodily capacities, with the introduction of new equipment for work, travel, and communication. It has changed radically in recent decades since the advent of computers and information technology, so much so that those individuals in their old age today find themselves in very different world from what they were born in and find hard to adjust to. We have greatly extended the range of our minds and senses through various news instruments and an ever-expanding media, making bodily skills less important and mental and social skills more crucial.

By way of travel and transportation, we can fly to distant countries in a matter of hours. We are now part of a mechanized society and spend most of our time working behind computers, even for our main means of communicating with other human beings. We cannot function without our cell phones and other high-tech equipment, which has become the focus of our attention and often tells us what to do and what we need to be informed about.

Our information technology enables us to communicate with people who may be in another country or continent, or who even may speak another language we do not know, which we get translated for us. Instead of traveling physically, we may travel by virtual reality, through a picture image of our face and physical body, not our actual physical presence.

Our virtual reality is becoming more important than our physical reality. We spend our time promoting that virtual reality, while we are confined in a room or sitting at a desk, constricted in our physical location, looking at a screen for our connection to the world as if the world itself was only virtual.

The ability to manipulate screens is becoming more important than our sensory capacities, whose acuity is getting diminished. We are becoming shadows of the screens we use, living in a two dimensional world defined by the media, lacking depth perception of nature or ourselves. We react to screens as if they were revealing the truth of the world of which they are merely a limited and transient appearance.

Altering our Physical Reality

If we look at our daily lives today, we see that we are seldom fixed in our local physical reality as defining who we are or what we are doing. Our consciousness is rarely focused directly on our bodies, but functions more through our mind and senses, extending to social influences and the media far removed from us, in which we may be anonymous. Through the media we may be concerned about global events, natural disasters, political changes in other countries, or famous personalities that would not have been known to those in previous non-technical societies. We can access various forms of communication from different places and countries, linking us to different social orders and their contrary considerations.

Though we are still identified with our physical bodies as who we are, we are more defined by our social image, which is more a media production than who we actually are. It is more important for us how we are seen by the media rather than who we actually are when we are alone and by ourselves. Our entertainment industry is often a realm of animation, fantasy or computer games that are removed from any physical reality. Such virtual reality creates a different mindset that removes us from our bodies but doesn't connect us to our inner Self either.

People today are willing to physically alter their bodies to make it more socially attractive, or to assume the social image they would like to have. This extends to plastic surgery, hormones, and many types of new drugs, which are now available. Similarly, we alter our outer reality from what it was during earlier humanity rooted in the world of nature to a high-tech urban environment, a world of equipment in which the human element is diminishing.

Similarly, we are willing to alter our minds to become more socially successful through various equipment and therapies, such as the use of special mind-altering and pain-relieving drugs. We change our physical appearance as necessary to make us more important in the eyes of others. We create an altered media image for ourselves, with special pictures or statements from us that have been altered by the media.

Indeed, we could say that our social identity, which is more extensive in time and space, is more important than our physical identity in the place where we reside. We rarely show other people who we physically are, which is seldom ideal, but prefer to appear how and when we would like others to see us, whatever acting or media manipulation it may require distorting who we really are.

Of course, this pursuit of social status has existed as long as our species, but today we have high tech tools to promote or change our social identity that go far beyond what previous generations had access to. Yet this also suggests to us is that we are not so fixated on our physical identity as we are using it as a tool for desires existing in the mind or even coming from the outside.

Our Physical Body as our Point Focus, Greater Reality of the Mind

The fact is that the physical body has become but a local point focus for a non-local reality defined more by our technology, media, and our minds. We don't want to be limited to our physical body or its place in which we reside. We want to be free to travel and experience the entire world, or just see it on a screen. While we must take care of the bodily focus of our lives, it is merely the launching pad for the pursuit of a greater social reality we don't yet understand.

This means that we don't believe we are simply physical beings, but rather that we are social and mental beings capable of expanding our boundaries to yet more subtle realities and experiences. We depend upon the body for our mortal existence, but our desires can go far beyond it.

To be trapped in physical restrictions, as confined to a bed or a wheelchair is not desirable for us. We value the body not just in itself but as a vehicle for broader range of travel, communication, action and entertainment defined by the mind and the mental ego.

If you look deeply into your life experience, you will see that you don't believe you are simply a physical being, a collection of organs, tissues, or biological functions. You have a physical body but you use it to benefit the desires of your mind and your interests in many aspects of society, life and the world.

Our minds can explore history, imagine the future, learn about the structure of the cosmos, or contemplate the origins of time and space. Our minds have access to realities beyond the body, at least by way of thought. The mind has realms of philosophy, psychology, cosmology and spirituality to pursue, not just biological necessities, though these may be woven together.

At a philosophical level, our minds can contemplate eternal verities and abstract thoughts that transcend any physical correlate, whether truth, being, the eternal or the infinite, or the laws of the universe overall. While this is largely speculative it does reflect higher capacities that we can develop, such as the practice of meditation that is becoming widely used.

At an artistic level, our minds can experience lasting or eternal beauty through various harmonious forms, expressions and arrangements, whether in poetry and literature, painting and sculpture, music and dance, drama or tragedy, which can be purely imaginary. We are looking to grasp an essence behind appearances, starting with that of our own body, and not just satisfied with what we or the world appear to be at an outer sensory level.

At a religious level, our minds can conceive of something infinite, eternal, Divine, heavenly worlds, some higher soul or spirit, ritual, theology or mysticism, which can become the basis of our deepest emotions and beliefs that we are even willing to die for. Or we can become aware of the sacred nature of all life with spirits or subtle energies everywhere, as commonly occurs when we commune with nature. We live in a world of energy, information, and intelligence, not just a bodily reality.

At a yogic level, we can read about the lives and teachings of great gurus and sages and partake of their wisdom, experience, and realization, including the higher states of Samadhi in which their consciousness can reach the highest bliss and awareness beyond all limitations of body and mind. This is in fact our most direct means of going beyond physical and socially-constructed reality.

Indeed, our minds are by nature more subtle, malleable, and changeable than our bodies, having a greater scope of awareness in time and space. The mind can regard the body as an instrument of its own knowing and feeling, but it can also see the body as a burden, preventing the fulfillment of our mental aspirations by drawing us down into physical needs and compulsions, even debilitating diseases, and of course death in the end. The mind can imagine a new or better body to develop or to aspire to. The mind can even go against the nature of the body, wanting to achieve or express something the body may not enjoy.

Let us not forget that a third of our lives is passed in state of sleep in which we withdraw from our physical identity and action altogether, and even withdraw from the mind in the state of deep sleep. Our daily experience is not entirely physical, but our physical experience is put into a state of hiatus or withdrawal every day. The body is not the whole of our life and experience but only the material foundation that we easily forget.

The idea of a transcendent Self-realization as in Yoga and Vedanta is something within the range of our thought, though we may be very far from realizing or even conceiving it. None of us want to die, which is the ultimate end of the physical body, so there is evidence that there is something deep within us beyond the body and the temporal world which even science today may not understand. The fact is that we are all looking for a higher consciousness beyond physical and social constraints, however vaguely we may formulate it, only imagine, or speculate about it. We do not want to be confined to the limitations of the body or its eventual death.

Please remember this ability of your mind to look beyond physical reality, even beyond mental reality as we know it. Remember our current information technology as taking you into a virtual reality beyond physical reality that consists of more energy and information than physical form.

Yet there are yet more subtle realities in the higher mind that transcends technology as we know it, the mind as part of a yogic spirituality rooted in a consciousness beyond the time and space. So,

33

neither body nor mind are final for us. We can look beyond the outer mind and its limited vision to a higher awareness in which the mind is also perceived as heavy, dense and limited like the body to which it remains attached.

We have an intuitive sense of an awareness beyond the thought-based mind. We easily tire of our mind's uncertainties, insecurities, doubts, worries, fears and desires. A sense of something transcendent is inherent within us, noticeable even in the dreams and fantasies of childhood, and longed for again as our body grows older. That search for transcendence can take us to our true Self or Atman that we must all eventually aspire to in order to go beyond death and sorrow.

We all have the sense of an inner reality beyond the body and mind and beyond our outer personality and the material world. Exploring that is the basis of Self-examination and Self-inquiry in Vedanta. The pursuit of Self-realization has a crucial place in our evolving high tech society that is looking beyond physical limitations to an understanding of the universe as a whole. We must recognize that out sense of self is a work in process with many higher potentials that we are just beginning to imagine, including beyond body and mind.

The quest for Self-realization requires a radical shift in how we live and how we view ourselves, transcending our views of time, place, and person. It requires that we embrace the consciousness in the universe as our true nature, which transcends all technology, not that we make our technology an end in itself. We are not a body, a machine, a computer or virtual reality, we are the Seer of all.

The true Self is nothing artificial, contrived, constructed, manmade or machine-made. It is not a product of time, circumstances or situations, or the opinions and judgements of others. In fact, it is the witness of all externality extending to body and mind, as mere changing phenomena, while its inner awareness is beyond time, space and person. So let us look deeper than virtual or imagined reality, to the eternal reality of our own inner Being.

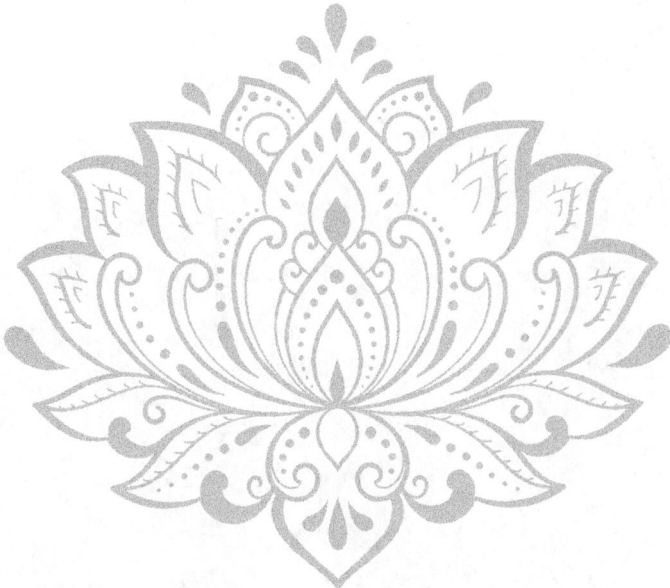

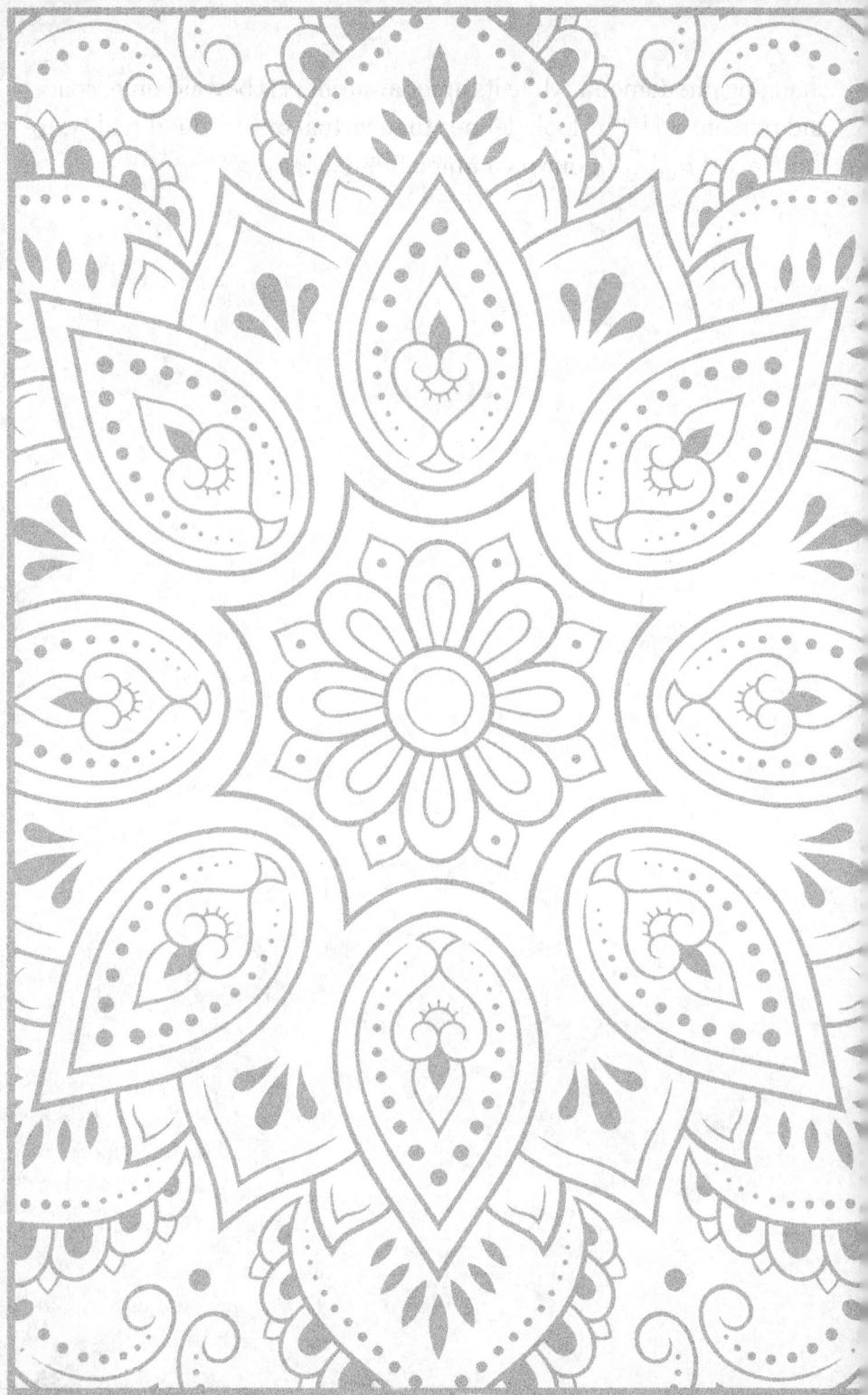

1.4

Self (Atman), *Brahman* and Ishvara

Self-realization is associated with God-realization or realization of the Divine in various Yoga traditions, particularly in modern times relative to a western audience. In Sanskrit Self-realization is the realization of the Atman or the Supreme Self (Paramatman), the Self of all. It is associated with realization of *Brahman*, the Supreme Reality. Yet to understand this we must first understand what Brahman refers to.

Brahman is said to be the supreme reality, beyond time, space and karma, all creatures and worlds known or unknown, manifest or unmanifest. It is defined in terms of Being-Consciousness-Bliss Absolute or *Satchidananda*: eternal being and truth (Sat), infinite consciousness (Chit), and complete and unbroken bliss (Ananda). Brahman and Atman are one. The experience of that as one's true nature is Self-realization.

Brahman is the foundation and origin of the manifest universe, but in its own nature is transcendent to any manifestation, which but waves on its boundless ocean. Brahman is beyond name, form, number, and person, beyond anything that can be cognized or thought of as an object. Brahman is the substratum and underlying reality of everything but is not itself subject to any change, division, or differentiation. Everything arises from it, but it is not limited by anything.

Brahman is the Absolute of Vedantic philosophy, the supreme principle at the root of all existence. Brahman is one only and non-dual (Advaita). There is nothing outside of it. Everything in essence is Brahman, however diverse the outer appearances. Brahman is the cosmic reality, the universal being, but extends beyond these to the unmanifest and unknowable by the mind.

Yoga-Vedanta equates Atman and Brahman, as our inmost Self and the Transcendent Reality. It means that you, the individual being, is in essence God or the Divine, though understood according to these Vedantic terms. This is quite a remarkable statement that has no simple correspondence in western philosophy or modern science. The inmost core of our Being and Self-awareness is not only one with the Divine as the Cosmic creative intelligence and force, but also one with the Transcendent Reality beyond all possible realms of manifestation or universes. This is unique in the spiritual and mystical philosophies and theologies of the world.

Meaning of *Brahman* and *Ishvara*

Brahman like Atman is a difficult term to translate and has no easy or complete equivalent in western philosophy or theology. Brahman is sometimes referred to as God or as the Godhead. Brahman is the origin and end of all. It is the material and efficient cause of the universe. Yet Brahman also transcends any creation or Creator as usually described in western philosophy or theology. Brahman is impersonal but is the substratum of all Consciousness through which a personal deity can arise.

God or the Divine as the Universal Creator is sometime called Brahman with qualities or *Saguna Brahman*, as contrasted to Brahman without qualities or *Nirguna Brahman*. This Universal Creator is called *Ishvara* in Vedic philosophy, which means the ruling power behind the three forces of the creation, preservation and dissolution of the universe, the Divine as the causal or guiding intelligence behind the universe in its manifestation.

Ishvara, however, is an inner reality, the Divine with us and the Self of the universe, not a deity apart from us or apart from the universe. Ishvara is not a God separate from its creation which is its Self-manifestation. Ishvara is the underlying intelligence that guides and shapes the universe but as an expression of itself, the universal or cosmic Guru.

Ishvara is one of the key terms of Bhakti Yoga or the Yoga of Devotion as in "Ishvara Pranidhana" of the Yoga Sutras, surrender to the Divine as the guiding intelligence within us. Ishvara has a personal aspect as representing manifest consciousness overall, through which the process of embodiment occurs.

Yet Ishvara is not like the human person, but is the Supreme Person, like Sri Krishna as Purushottama. Ishvara can be described in biological terms as male or female, though it transcends both. Generally, Ishvara is regarded metaphorically as masculine but its power and expression is feminine, Ishvari or Shakti. As such, it is best to use the term Ishvara directly and not reduce it to other theological traditions that have a different view of our true Self, the Universal Deity, and the cosmic reality.

Ramana Maharshi and Belief in God

Ramana Maharshi did not emphasize the term God even for his western disciples. When asked, how does one know God? Ramana replied that God is a distant entity, so it is best to leave God out of the pursuit of the Supreme Truth. It is better to inquire into oneself, if one knows one's Self, one knows God. If one knows God but does not know one's Self, such a deity is not the ultimate truth but an imagination of the mind.

As such, Advaita (Non-dualism) and Self-realization are relevant for those who may not have devotion to a personal God, are part of any formal religious tradition, or have any religious belief, who may even consider themselves to be Agnostics or Atheists. A religious belief, particularly if it is exclusive in nature, can be an obstacle along the path of Self-realization.

Yet Advaita Vedanta does honor the path of devotion or Bhakti Yoga as a path in its own right, leading us inward to our true Self that is the Self of all the Devatas or deity forms, which are viewed as manifestations of our true Self. We see this in Ramana's devotion to Shiva Mahadeva and in Shankaracharya's powerful mantric hymns (stotras) to the Hindu deities. Such Bhakti or devotion is a Yoga or path of Sadhana (spiritual practice) and meditation. It is not just a faith or belief that is required but a surrender inwardly to the Divine within us, which is beyond any beliefs of the mind.

Ramana Maharshi refers to the Creator (Ishvara) and to various aspects of Devotion and Karma Yoga in his teachings for different types of aspirants. The Vedantic view is that the same Self and Being (Atman) is present both in Ishvara (Cosmic Self) and the Jivatman (Individual Self), which represent the collective and individual aspects of the universal manifestation. Knowing the Self, one knows and is Brahman and is one with Ishvara as well.

The Advaitic path is to inquire within oneself to discover one's true nature as pure consciousness, to make Self-knowledge the supreme principle, not knowledge of the outer world, the mind or even knowledge of subtle worlds. Through the Self, your true nature, Ishvara and Brahman are known in their underlying unity beyond name and form as one with your own essence of Being. The Divine as Ishvara and devotion to Ishvara as a path of Bhakti Yoga are important. In fact, as the Cosmic Intelligence, Ishvara is the Adi-Guru, the original Guru of the universe as noted in the *Yoga Sutras*.

Knowledge of Being (*Sadvidya*)

Ramana composed another important Sanskrit work called *Saddarshana* or "Knowledge of Being," which along with *Upadesha Saram* discussed in this book are his two main texts. This reflects the knowledge of Being or Sadvidya of the *Upanishads*, notably the *Chhandogya*.

Being or *Sat* is the key term for defining Brahman, which is beyond any particularized manifestation, action, or definition. We are all present in that oneness of Being which is behind and beyond all time and space, birth and death. Our manifest world is a realm of becoming, which rests upon this immutable Being. Everything changes at every second and is ultimately impermanent and momentary. That pure Being is the presence of Consciousness beyond the mind.

Self-knowledge is synonymous with Knowledge of Being (Atma Vidya is Sadvidya). Dwelling in pure Being takes us into Atman and Brahman as one. That pure Being is the basis of our inmost identity, awareness, and happiness.

Realization of Atman and realization of Brahman are equivalent, the same essence of Being in the individual and in the universe. Unity with God, or communion with God can have different meanings in different theologies, most of which do not have a concept of God-realization, just as they do not have a concept of the Supreme Self. We must understand Self-realization in this Vedantic philosophy for clarity about its teachings.

Advaitic texts are not so much concerned about the semantic details of theology, but about understanding how our own minds work and removing all illusion and ignorance from our thoughts. Advaita holds that the supreme truth and reality is Self-effulgent. It shines forth of its own accord once we remove ignorance and attachment from our own minds.

That is why Advaita texts like Shankara's *Vivekachudamani* for example, contain little of metaphysics but go into detail about the proper purification of the mind and emotions (chitta-shuddhi, chitta-prasadana). We must possess the necessary awareness for Self-inquiry to be possible and not just an imagination of the mind still caught in ignorance.

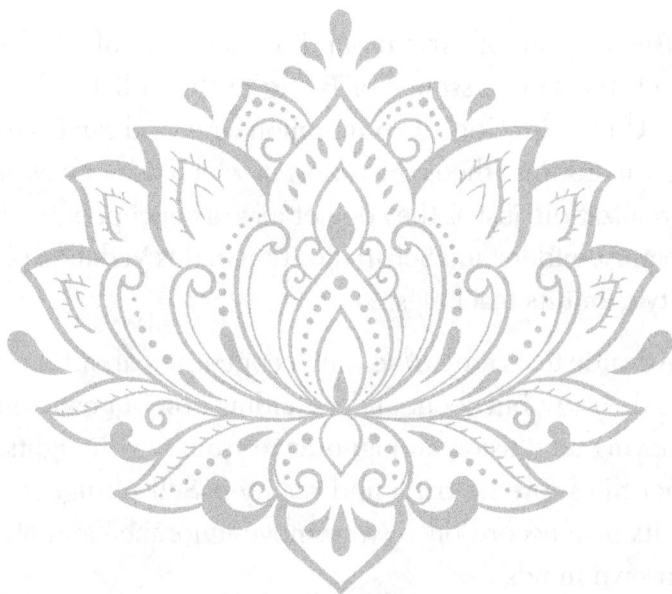

1.5

The Paths of Yoga and the Yoga of Knowledge

Yoga is often defined as a way of Self-Realization, God-Realization or Cosmic Consciousness which are frequently equated but can have different meanings. The realization of the Supreme Self, Atman, or Purusha is emphasized in Yoga texts like *Yoga Sutras*, *Bhagavad Gita*, and many Yoga texts as the goal of Yoga.

Yoga has many traditional paths of Yoga over its thousands of years all of which aim at Self-realization of which five are most important:

1. **Jnana Yoga or the Yoga of Knowledge,** as defined in Advaita Vedanta. Its goal is Self-realization as realization of the Atman or inmost Self of all, as in the teachings of Ramana and Shankaracharya (Adi Shankara). Jnana Yoga or the Yoga of Knowledge is often regarded as the highest of the Yogas as it can directly take up to the highest Self-realization.

    Yet it is the most difficult of the Yoga paths at it requires a discerning intelligence and tremendous detachment to realistically pursue, which is extremely rare at all times, and more so today for our sensate and materialistic culture, and egoistic mindset. Its main approach is through Self-inquiry and study of Vedantic texts, not through outer methods or techniques, though these may have some preliminary value.

2. **Bhakti Yoga or the Yoga of Devotion,** which has many deity lines like Shiva, Vishnu, Devi, Ganesha, and Surya in Hindu traditions. Its goal is mergence in the Divine as the Supreme Person (Purusha).

   Bhakti Yoga or the Yoga of Deotion generally consists of worship of the deity within us. Surrender, which is the highest approach of Bhakti Yoga, can also take us to Self-realization. Those who equate Self-realization and God-realization are usually looking at God or the Divine as the Self in all beings, the Ishvara of Yoga Sutras.

3. **Karma Yoga or the Yoga of Selfless Action,** which is usually connected to the teachings of Jnana or Bhakti as a preliminary practice to purify the mind. Karma Yoga as the Yoga of Action can take many forms, but it must rest internally on devotion or knowledge. It is not so much a separate Yoga path as a part of the other paths. One who cannot work selflessly cannot perform meditation or internal Yoga practices selflessly either.

   Karma Yoga includes the practices of Dharmic living to purify the mind as in the Yamas and Niyamas of Yoga, properly discharging one's duties in life. It includes the practice of ritual worship in all its forms. At the highest level, Karma Yoga includes performing our actions in life without a loss of Self-awareness, or devotion to the Divine as part of Jnana and Bhakti Yogas.

4. **Raja Yoga,** mainly the eightfold (ashtanga) approach of Patanjali's Yoga Sutras, emphasizes meditation and control of the mind to realize the Purusha or Atman through Samadhi, which is its main orientation. This means that Raja Yoga is close to Jnana Yoga as its goal is also the Self-realization by transcending the body and mind. It aims at

changes in attitude, values, perception, and awareness, not simply at external actions or techniques. Jnana Yoga and Vedanta provide the ultimate philosophy behind Raja Yoga, the nature of Atman, Purusha, and Ishvara.

5. **Hatha Yoga,** emphasizing the use of Prana through various techniques, with a notable place for asanas or yoga postures, is regarded as preliminary to Raja Yoga and realization of Purusha/Atman. Hatha Yoga emphasizes the use of Prana and Pranayama to calm and transcend the mind. Modern Hatha Yoga, we should note, is more of an asana approach, not the full field of Hatha Yoga. Hatha Yoga is often regarded as preliminary approach of purifying body and mind to develop the foundation to practice Raja Yoga or Jnana Yoga.

Today the physical aspect of Yoga is the most popular and definitive throughout the world as taught in group Yoga classes. Asana is what people mean by "doing Yoga", though that is not its traditional meaning. Its goal is physical health and fitness, extending to mental wellbeing, but not necessarily Self-realization, the true nature of which is rarely explained in depth in Yoga teacher training programs.

Yoga teacher's trainings aim at teaching how to guide asana classes, usually in specific sequences or routines. This means that the popular Yoga remains different from the traditional or spiritual Yoga relative to Self-realization in the Vedantic sense. This Asana Yoga serving to prepare the way for meditation and Self-inquiry, though cannot be equated with it.

To understand true Yoga and Self-realization, we must return Yoga to its traditional definition as a way of Self-knowledge (Atmavidya). This is what the original great Yoga Gurus who brought Yoga to the western world emphasized in their teachings, such as Swami Vivekananda, Swami Rama Tirtha, Paramahansa Yogananda,

YOGA BEYOND BODY & MIND | Frawley

Swami Sivananda of Rishikesh and Sri Aurobindo, among many others. Patanjali in *Yoga Sutras* refers to Yoga as the means of realizing the Purusha or Seer through transcending the mind (chitta) and its disturbances. This is the way of Self-realization beyond body and mind.

The Yoga of Knowledge (Jnana Yoga)

The Yoga of knowledge as taught in Advaita Vedanta is relevant to all Yogic paths, as it orients us to the highest goal of Yoga as Self-realization. Yet as one of the highest of the paths it may require proficiency in the lesser Yoga practices to effectively pursue it, meaning mastery of body and mind and transcendence of the ego.

Yoga rests upon a concept of proficiency called *adhikara* in Sanskrit as all disciplines tend to consider. For example, you can't teach someone how to run if they don't know how to walk. You can't teach someone poetry in a language they don't know. You can't ask someone to scale a high mountain if they have never climbed a small hill. Such insistence on right qualifications and right aptitude occurs in all human skills and professions and necessary to protect us from injury or errors.

Advaitic Sadhana or practice consists of two phases:

1. The first is purifying or making sattvic the body, prana, senses, and mind, with a pure and concentrated intelligence as the key. It means letting go of the ego and our sense of bodily identity.

2. The second is transcending the mind and its disturbances, going beyond the mind. The second step cannot be accomplished without the first as without a sattvic mind, our minds will be drawn back into agitation and inertia and cannot directly connect to the Self within.

While Self-inquiry (Atma-vichara) is the main approach for Self-realization, there are many aids for purifying the body and mind to make this possible. These include practices of the other Yogas like service, devotion, ritual, mantras, or pilgrimage. Study of Vedantic texts can also be part of this. They are the basis of the Yamas and Niyamas as discussed in *Yoga Sutras*. Asana, Pranayama and Pratyahara forming the outer Yoga have their main place here as well.

The Yoga of knowledge is born of the fire of *tapas*, concentrated Yoga practice, which is the root of all Yogic purification methods. This includes developing the patience, determination, and concentration necessary to master them mind. Self-inquiry requires an internal fire of consciousness or flame of awareness, the ultimate tapas. All negative thoughts and emotions must be offered into that inner fire for them to be removed, so that the light of Consciousness can shine forth without any obstruction or impurity. We must learn to offer our minds into the Agni or flame of awareness that is the Atman within, on which the *Vedas* were based.

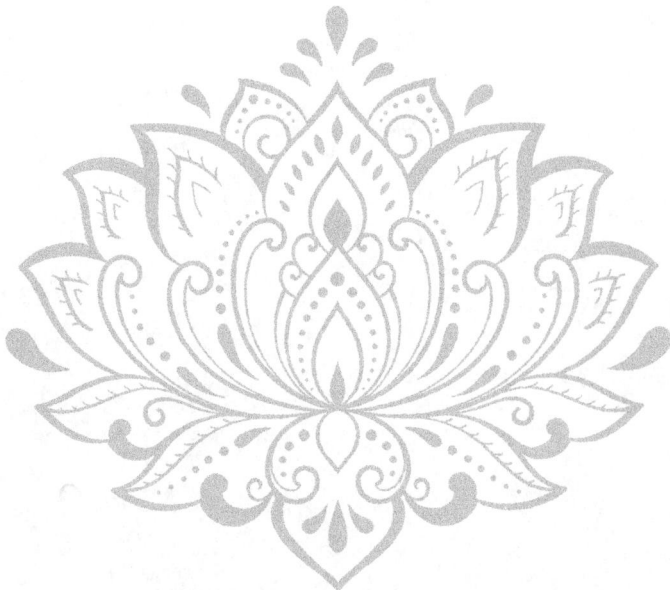

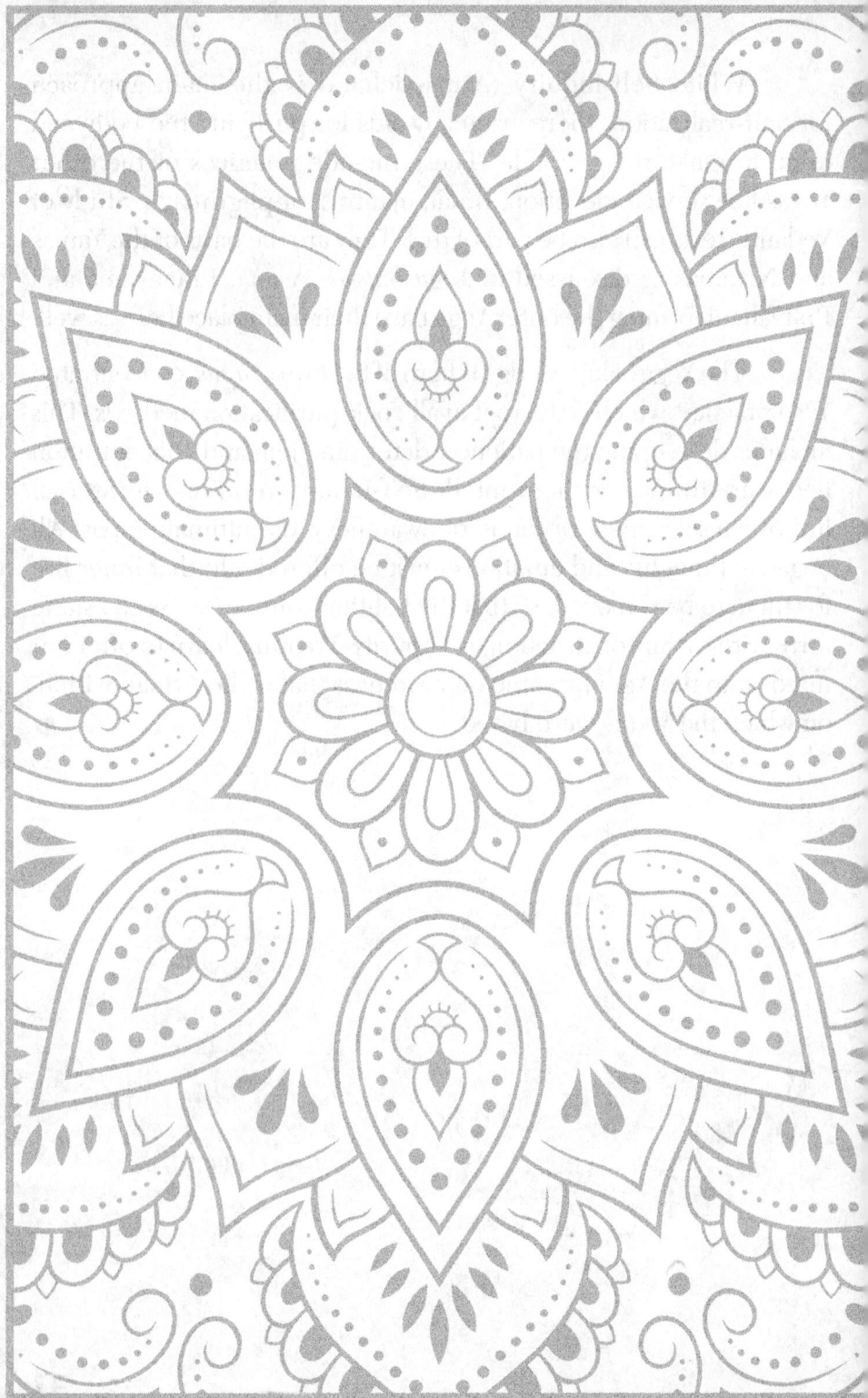

1.6
Meditation and Self-Inquiry
Dhyana and Vichara

An important issue in discussing profound teachings of higher states of consciousness which are explained in Sanskrit texts is that we rarely have equivalent terms in English to relate to these to or define them properly. Along with this, we find that many of these Sanskrit terms have become popularized in meanings which are limited or incorrect. While I have translated many Sanskrit terms in the current book, these translations are only approximate, and must be looked at in a deeper light which we have also tried to explain.

Meditation has become a common term in the world today. Many groups use it whether in different dharmic traditions, religions, or mystical teachings, even in psychology today. The importance of meditation was introduced into global discourse over the last century by gurus for the meditation practices of their students, but has spread into various discourses whether spiritual, academic, or even the mass culture.

Yet the term meditation as used in the English language today has a broad range of connotations for various meditation practices and techniques, including various types of prayer, contemplation, concentration, visualization, or imagination. Such various types of what is now called meditation may not be is not equivalent to *Dhyana* in Sanskrit or part of a Sadhana or yogic practice, of which there are many types.

Meditation as Dhyana in Sanskrit has a more specific meaning than meditation in common discussions today. It has connections to the other limbs of Yoga or the different branches of Yoga, mainly the Yoga of Knowledge. While meditation remains the best English equivalent to Dhyana in Sanskrit, it falls short of the inner meaning, or the different applications of Dhyana in Yoga and Vedanta traditions. Some of what may be called meditation in the West may not be called Dhyana in dharmic traditions as it may still be regarded as a mental activity.

Self-inquiry (Atma-Vichara) is the main practice followed in Advaita Vedanta. One could call it a type of meditation as it involves profound introspection extending to Samadhi, the Yogic state of unity Consciousness that arises through Dhyana. Yet the term used for it is not simply Dhyana or meditation in Vedanta but *Vichara*, which implies inquiry and examination.

Vichara implies a process of questioning, but as directed within, not the outer mechanical conditioned thought of the ordinary mind and its memory-based patterns and sensory reactions. Vichara requires questioning the mind itself and all its assumptions, activities and means of knowledge. *Atma-vichara* is an introspective inquiry, a self-observation, which requires a turning of the mind and prana within, which requires silencing the outer mind and its ego-based thoughts, desires, or assumptions.

As such, we can call Vichara as a meditative inquiry. It is not an outer inquiry using the senses, words, numbers, concepts or logics, or any type of mere information gathering. It requires progressively removing the veils of our thoughts to discover the light of Self-awareness, which provides light to the mind by way of reflection but inherently transcends it. Vichara can be guided or stimulated by the study of various Vedantic texts that teach its key principles and how to examine these in our mental activities overall, extending to the state o deep sleep.

However, there are forms of meditation, which are not a process of Vichara. These include passive forms of meditation, like meditating on a mantra, a yantra, a form, some aspect of nature, space, or the void etc. Yet these can be turned into a type of Vichara if we call up the questions Who am I during the meditation as "Who is meditating and what are the forms being meditated upon?"

Passive and reflective forms of meditation teach us that our minds will become immersed in whatever we give our primary attention to, particularly when they are in a concentrated and focused state. Vichara can be called a questioning type of meditation but only in the sense of focusing the mind in searching out its origin in Consciousness, a letting go of the mind and its identities, not an ordinary mental activity.

As Self-inquiry negates all thoughts and takes them back to their origin in the Self, it also involves a reduction of outer activity and any outer engagement or external identification with the mind and sense. It requires turning of the stream of the awareness within until it merges into the ocean of Consciousness, and the mind becomes no-mind.

Asking the Question, *"Who Am I?"*

Self-inquiry is rooted in asking the most fundamental of all questions, which is Who am I? and what is our true Self and real identity in the universe. Truly asking the question Who am I? is not a mere mental asking of the question, much less looking for our Self outwardly in the body or the external world. It is not the mind asking, "Who am I"? but questioning our mental and physical or mind-body identity, a rejection of all outer identifications. Its conclusion is not "I think therefore I am" of western philosophy which is only a projection of the mental self and its illusions. It is "I am, therefore, I think", which indicates our true I am exists before and beyond all thoughts and beyond the mind.

The meaning of "Who" in the question Who am I is not the who of the outer or social personality, a person with a name, occupation or location in time and space according to a physical body and various outer possessions. It is not the mental self defined by thought, but what thought cannot define. The question relates to the seer or observer of the movements of body and mind. Implies its capacity to transcend them in detached observation beyond any theory, belief, or conclusion of the mind.

One cannot just simply verbally ask the question Who Am I? and find out the core of one's being. That is little more than a mind game. It is like the inquiry of someone who has amnesia trying to discover who they really are. It must have an urgency and importance that can stop all other thoughts, interests, and desires. It implies that one has already rejected ones physical and mental identity as superficial or illusory and is looking for what is inherently beyond these. The question therefore is if I am not this body or mind than who or what am I, and how can I dwell in that inner reality while I function in this outer world?

True Self-realization is not simply a meditative state of mind, though that is helpful if not essential in bringing it about. It is the natural state of Consciousness (chit) beyond the individual mind (chitta/manas) and its functions which are but its instruments. In short, it is a state beyond the mind. It has been called a state of no-mind, though that must also be understood not as a lack of intelligence, discernment or focus. The Self is a state of pure awareness beyond the dualities and distractions of the thought based mind. It is a state of universal and transcendent awareness beyond the individualized or embodied mind and all its compulsions, needs and disturbances. It takes us to an entirely different state of consciousness in which the mind is but a shadow or reflection.

Neti Neti, the Path of Negation

Self-inquiry is part of a path of negation, discarding or letting of all that is not-Self as unreal or irrelevant. It asks us to question every thought or emotion that comes up in the mind, along with the motivation which drives it. Whatever thought arises in the mind is not who we really are as the witness or seer of the mind. It is some stimulation, compulsion or reaction from the outside, from other people or physical involvements. All thoughts, including relative to our personal identity, can be negated or removed as not-Self, not who we truly are, but only part of our outer expression or the outer world. We must learn to reject our thoughts as "I am not this" and "this is not mine." All these thoughts in any case will disappear in the movement of time.

Self-realization is gained by calming, silencing, negating, detaching or disidentification with the mind, which the Yoga Sutras teaches as *Nirodha*, removing us from considering the functions of the mind (chitta vrittis) as belonging to us or defining who we truly are. We can then witness the mind and use it as a practical instrument for our outer life, but not as the truth of our immortal nature, or the means of knowing the ultimate reality beyond birth and death.

Self-realization relates to the eighth and foundation limb of Yoga, which is Samadhi, the state of unitary awareness. Self-realization is the highest samadhi of resting in one's true nature beyond all the disturbances of the mind. This samadhi of the Self rests upon a one-pointed mind and a unified mental field in which we ultimately let go of the mind and its actions as unreal.

Samadhi is defined twofold in yogic texts as *savikalpa* and *nirvikalpa*, with or without mental movements, motivations or imaginations (vikalpa). Self-realization is equated with Nirvikalpa Samadhi, which no thought can influence, limit or define, and which continues as our natural state of pure awareness.

Self-realization is the natural state of the Purusha or Atman beyond the gunas or qualities of nature as sattva, rajas and tamas, which means beyond chitta or mind in which the gunas operate. This state is also called *Sahaja Samadhi* or the natural Samadhi. It is not an ordinary state of mind, but the pure consciousness beyond the mind, which we can only access through the silent mind when the mind becomes no mind.

Self-realization and Silence

Self-realization as the Supreme Reality of Brahman is beyond all concepts and beliefs, where speech and mind turn back unable to reach, as the *Upanishads* teach. Words and ideas are but indicators not the reality itself. As such, Advaita is beyond all philosophy and logic or science. Realization of the Self occurs in when one is no longer drawn into the compulsions and illusions of the mind, where no words or numbers can enter, when thought and the mind fall silent. It a change of being to a higher dimension of awareness beyond all that is limited.

Bhagavan Ramana Maharshi emphasizes that inner silence as the highest truth. This is the silence of the spiritual heart (Hridaya) in which the Divine Self eternally dwells at the core of our being like a hidden flame. Communication from the spiritual heart is a heart-to-heart teaching, not in an emotional sense, but abiding at the core of our being beyond body and mind, which is the highest teaching. If you can realize your essential being, there is no need to talk about it as something apart from you, which all words, names and concepts imply.

All discussion ends in this supreme silence which is the vibratory essence behind the universe and our own awareness pervading all space. Let us be open to that inner silence of Self-realization, not as just a mental discipline but as the highest state of peace or shanti within us and in the entire universe.

Certainly, teachings, mantras and insights can guide us in that direction, removing the deep-seated attachments and conditioning of the mind. But that inner stillness and silence abides in state of Samadhi, the unitary and silent awareness that is Self-illuminating, Self-revealing and ever overflowing.

May we come to rest in the light of that boundless Self-awareness for which entire universes are but bubbles on its endless sea, which extends beyond anything that can be described, known, or imagined. Let us forget outer quantities and appearances and embrace the highest state of pure Being ever at peace within itself but also overflowing into boundless creativity without losing itself.

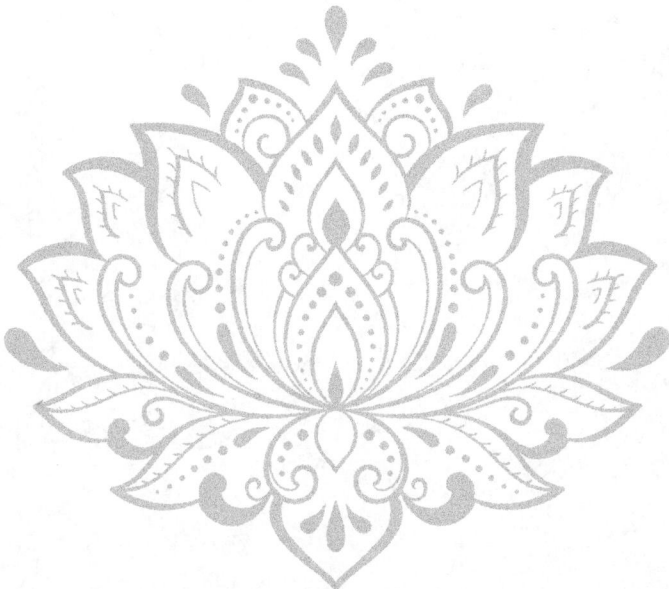

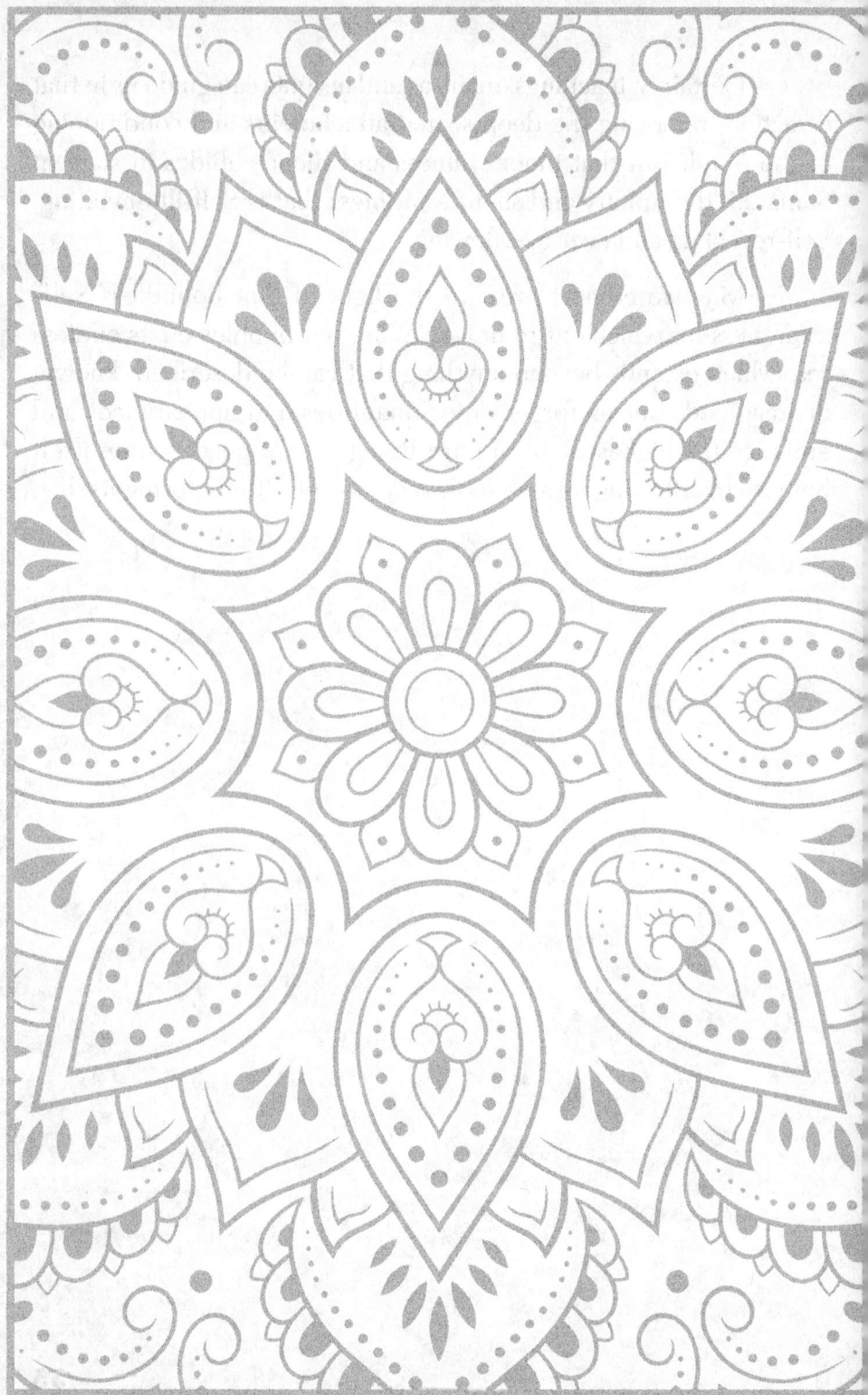

1.7
Advaita, Neo-*Advaita*, and Yoga

It is sometimes stated that there is no path to Self-realization and non-duality because the Self (Atman) is your true nature, as such it is always present, compared to which there is no second entity, no other. The Self is not something new to be achieved but only a recognition of what we already are and have always been at the core of our being, but what in our ignorance we have forgotten and covered over with outer fears and desires.

Sometimes the metaphor of the "ten men" is used to explain this. A group of ten men goes off on a long journey and one by one the men return. Then the leader of the group counts off the returning members and only finds nine, which makes him worry about the tenth person who was lost and wants to go and find him as well. Then he recognizes that he forgot to count himself and he himself is the tenth man! and the imaginary loss disappears, much to his relief.

We forget to count our true Self or remember our true nature, and so there is a false sense of loss or non-accomplishment and seeking to regain what we already are. This is the illusion of the search for the Self, as we in truth are that Self. Yet truly recognizing that is not a mental recognition but a realization in our inmost awareness.

The way to the Self is to return to the essence of our being. There is another anecdote about Ramana Maharshi in this regard. A seeker came to him and explained all the different spiritual paths he has already followed and that, sadly, he still has not reached his goal. He then asks Ramana which path he should follow to finally reach his goal. Ramana smiling replied that he should go back the way that he came, meaning to return to his true nature and give up the illusory seeking of the mind.

We are all inherently Self-realized at the core of our being, though not in our ordinary mind and ego. What is required is removing the ignorance, the lack of Self-knowledge, which obscures it, like the clouds can obscure our view of the sun in the sky but not the sun itself.   This return to the immortal Self is not an easy process as our ego and bodily identity has been formed throughout many lifetimes and is shaped by our education and reinforced by our society. For a person still trapped in the ego-mind to claim to be Self-realized because that is our true nature is an illusion that prevents any deeper realization. A determined Self-inquiry is required to remove the identification with body and mind, not just mental idea that all are Self-realized.

Unfortunately, it is convenient to the ego to claim to be a spiritual master or guru, which allows a person to gather wealth, power, and followers, affording them greater enjoyment and adulation. That is why among public teachers of the higher knowledge there can distortions and an exaggerated ego. The nature of the ego is wishful thinking, and to become recognized as Self-realized, even though one is not, is a great temptation for the ego, particularly at a mental level. It is to become a God for others without any real inner transformation.

To call ourselves Self-realized when we are still caught up in the ego-mind is a deception that prevents any real progress. Humility is the basis of Self-knowledge, which begins when we recognize that we really do not know who we are and that our bodily and mental identity is an outer illusion, not an inner reality. Until we learn to deeply examine and question the mind and all of its deep-seated forms of wishful thinking, we have not yet entered the real way of Self-realization.

Who is Self-realized?

Who then is Self-realized in this supreme sense of the term, realization of Paramatman, the Supreme Self-awareness behind all existence? What person can we say is actually Self-realized? As Self-realization is beyond time, place and person, name and form, body, and mind, it is difficult to say if a person is Self-realized, or if such a statement has any real meaning at all.

What we see as a person is their physical body in a certain outer context not their inner being. We may study their words and teachings. We may recognize their name or face or know some details of their personal life. Yet their inner state of awareness is not directly known to us. Different human being can have different degrees of charisma, intelligence, devotion, or wisdom and still not be dwelling in that highest Self-realization.

When a person wakes up from a dream, we don't say that the dreamer has continued his dream life in the waking state, but that the illusory dream and the dreamer have disappeared, and the waking self has returned to its own waking reality. Nor can someone in a dream state be asked to identify who in their dream is actually awake and not sleeping?

If we say that Ramana Maharshi or some other guru has achieved Self-realization it can create misconceptions, as Ramana himself noted, never claiming to be uniquely realized as a person. Ramana never encouraged people to adulate him or any other person as the supreme Self. He never claimed to have founded a new religion in his name, to have developed a new Yoga technique for everyone, or to have any unique Divine dispensation of his own as a new messenger of God.

Ramana lived humbly and simply, owning only a few loin cloths. He did not travel and teach or establish any institution in his name. He did have close disciples, who stayed in his presence to imbibe his teachings inherent. He looked upon all as a spiritual father. He directed everyone to their highest truth and gave them practical guidance in their sadhana.

Ramana did not formally take on the orange robes of a monk or Sannyasi. Yet he did honor the traditional teachings of Advaita Vedanta, its great gurus, books and ashrams. He recommended and commented upon Vedantic teachings, including from the *Bhagavad Gita*, the works of Shankaracharya (Adi Shankara) and Advaitic texts like *Tripura Rahasya* or *Advaita Bodha Deepika*. In short, he was a teacher in the tradition of Advaita Vedanta, not apart from it.

The Self-realized guru is not a physical being or a particular body or face that we can see in person or in a picture. The true guru reflects a state of consciousness revealed in the teachings that they give, but only if we understand these at the core of our being. These teachings are not verbal or conceptual, they occur at a mind-to-mind and heart-to-heart level, and ultimately not as personal communication but as a realization of the Infinite and Eternal Self of all.

Neo-*Advaita* and Non-duality

Neo-Advaita is a term used for contemporary movements that focus on non-duality but without specifically following the tradition of Advaita Vedanta. They commonly emphasize a kind of instant enlightenment for all. Such teachings could be called "Advaita or Non-duality without Vedanta", as it does not include an indepth study of Advaita Vedanta through traditional texts and teachers. They often dismiss the Advaitic tradition of preparing the student by extensive training, service, study of texts, mantra, pranayama, and meditation. They can promote a kind of wishful thinking that anyone can claim to be Self-realized as a conclusion of the mind.

This New-Advaita or new Non-duality movement focuses on a few teachers, who may be from various traditions, but who usually appear as rebels outside of any formal tradition, following their own path more than a set tradition or lineage. As such, these teachings can appeal to those who are individualistic and do not want to be confined to any tradition, particularly from the past or from other cultures.

The teachings of Ramana Maharshi can appeal to them for the directness and simplicity of his approach. Though they may claim to be Ramana's followers, they may not have any specific connection to the greater tradition he was part of. They may go against the traditional rules of self-discipline of the Advaita Vedanta.

They may have little regard for any tradition, seeing non-duality as beyond any tradition, even beyond any pre-requisites of purification of body or mind and sattvic living. They may claim a direct transmission or direct realization, achieving Self-realization in a short period of time. They view Non-duality more as a modern global movement than any specific tradition. They may include Vedantic teachings like that of Ramana Maharshi along with other spiritual traditions or along with teachers outside of any tradition, adding aspects modern psychology, like Jungian, and quantum physics and its search for a field of consciousness behind the universe.

They may include Buddhist teachings, like Zen or Tibetan Buddhism, but as in the case of Advaita Vedanta, not formally follow or represent it. Some connect to the teachings of J. Krishnamurti who rejected the Vedantic tradition at a formal level of the Atman, though he often had similar approaches and teachings of his own.

This new Non-duality may connect all traditions or teachings that emphasize some form of unity consciousness or non-duality, which cuts across many religious and mystical traditions. It is often a diverse, variable, syncretic contemporary intellectual movement, but not a way of Self-realization beyond mind and ego. Some of its teachers claim they have gained enlightenment or Self-realization but have no traditional recognition for what they have accomplished.

The main danger in Neo-Advaitic groups and modern non-dualism is the idea that one can achieve instant enlightenment without any extensive preparation or sadhana, that following a tradition is not necessary, nor any formal practice required, even a guru being unnecessary. The idea they project is that anyone can achieve Self-realization immediately by just being told and accepting that one is Self-realized by nature, without any practice or sadhana required. Some would dispense with a living guru follow self-appointed or self-proclaimed gurus outside any formal tradition or lineage.

Ramana Maharshi in his *Upadesha Saram* notes there are different levels and aptitudes (adhikaras) of aspirants, and different teachings and stages of practice accordingly. He emphasizes that only a ripe or sattvic mind (pakva chitta), meaning a purified mind, can authentically approach Self-inquiry at an experiential level. For a mind caught in rajas and tamas, the factors of agitation and ignorance, to claim to be following or teaching Self-realization is wishful thinking or a mind game.

There are also many higher states of consciousness or simply unusual experiences between the ordinary state of the human mind and the highest Self-realization that may be mistaken for a true realization. Yoga teachings speak of many transient or illusory samadhis for example. A mind untrained in Yoga is especially vulnerable to these. There are similarly many drug-based experiences which are like transient Samadhis that can give rise to such illusions in the mind.

Advaita Vedanta and *Yoga Sutras*

Some proponents of Yoga do claim to teach Self-realization at least as the goal of Yoga. Most of the Yoga today is asana-based and meditation is a sidelight. Yet anyone who studies the *Yoga Sutras* seriously will see that Self-realization (realization of the Purusha) is the goal of the Yoga practice or Sadhana, not any physical postures.

Advaitic texts commonly incorporate the eight limbs of Yoga as mentioned in Patanjali's *Yoga Sutras*, and give this great value, both for purifying the body and mind and for transcending body and mind. For example, *Vivekachudamani* of Shankara does this. Advaitic texts also explain the Samadhis of Yoga, up to the highest state of Kaivalya., which they identify with Self-realization in the Advaitic text.

We must remember that most of the great gurus who brought Yoga to the West taught Yoga-Vedanta and many were Swamis in Vedantic orders. These include Swami Vivekananda and Ramakrishna Yoga-Vedanta, Paramahansa Yogananda and the main disciples of Swami Sivananda of Rishikesh, and followers of various Shankaracharyas and Vedantic Swamis, including Maharishi Mahesh Yogi.

Yet some scholars note that Advaitic texts going back to Adi Shankara do criticize Samkhya-Yoga philosophy in a few areas, though not in the main portion of their teachings. This has caused some people to think that Yoga and Vedanta are different and not compatible. Let us examine these areas in which Vedantins criticize Samkhya-Yoga, mainly certain views of the Samkhya system.

Advaitins like Shankara criticize Samkhya-Yoga as dualistic as the system states that Purusha and Prakriti are both eternal and different independent principles, constituting a kind of ultimate duality. Advaita Vedanta regards Prakriti as Maya or illusion which does not have any separate reality of its own, and so not constituting any ultimate duality.

63

Yet if we take a deep look at the Samkhya system, it states that the Purusha is the only independent and consciousness principle, while Prakriti is dependent and not-consciousness. This raises the question: How can a dependent and unconscious principle have any separate reality of its own? Obviously, it cannot. A dependent unconscious principle has no reality or awareness of its own. In other words, the very logic of Samkhya leads us to Advaita.

Advaitins also criticize Samkhya for its view that Purushas are many, which promotes another form of dualism. In the Advaitic system there is only One Self, Atman or Purusha in all beings. A multiplicity of Purushas only exists relative to embodied Purusha or Jivatman, not the realized Self but the ego caught in the process of karma and rebirth.

Samkhya states that the many Purushas do experience a common Prakriti or world of nature. The Purushas also have common powers and consist of pure consciousness, like a common genus but different species. Yet if the same Prakriti is common to all Purushas, need the Purushas be different?

Advaita states the Purusha is beyond the realm of name, form and number which is the domain of Prakriti. Samkhya also states that name and form belong to Prakriti not to the Purusha. As such, how can Purushas be counted, and relative to what other reality?

To differentiate between Purushas in any ultimate sense, to give them some numerical quantity appears contrary to the view of Samkhya that Purushas are inherently beyond Prakriti. Prakriti can be quantified but Purusha as beyond Prakriti is beyond all multiplicity and duality. What consists of pure consciousness only and is the seer of all quantities and appearances cannot itself be quantified.

Though the *Yoga Sutras* is traditionally connected to Samkhya, we also see much in the text that can be connected to Advaita and has been by many Advaitic gurus. The Kaivalya of the *Yoga Sutras* is connected to the Moksha of Advaita and its Nirvikalpa Samadhi. Meanwhile other Yoga texts, including the *Hatha Yoga Pradipika*, identify Samadhi, the highest state of Yoga with Advaita or Non-duality, showing that these differences have long been questioned.

My point here is not to get the reader involved in subtle philosophical debates but to point out that the *Yoga Sutras* have been and can still be used in the context of Advaita Vedanta, but only if it is not connected with certain dualistic positions of the Samkhya System which are questionable anyone. Such dualistic views do not seem necessary if the true goal of Yoga is Self-realization and unity with all.

Yet we must also remember that the highest Samadhi and Self-realization is beyond all words and concepts, so any formal or systematic philosophical explanation of it must be limited and eventually put aside for the direct experience in Samadhi of the beyond the mind state. As the minds of living beings are different, and as the Self is beyond the mind, all mental explications of the Self and Non-duality must at best be preparatory in nature and eventually be set aside like the raft that is left behind when one reaches the other shore. So let us not fight over mere semantics or logic but dive into that inner Self that no name, idea or number can limit or define.

Advaita Vedanta and the Yoga of the *Bhagavad Gita*

Yoga is a term with several applications in Sanskrit and various Yoga traditions. The Yoga Sutras are part of these, but there many others. The prime text on both Yoga and Vedanta is the same, the *Bhagavad Gita* of Sri Krishna.

Sri Krishna is the Yogavatara or avatar of Yoga. He is Yogeshvara or the lord of Yoga. Each chapter of the Gita is related to a certain type or knowledge of Yoga. Yoga permeates the entire text, its topics, and teachings.

Sri Krishna states that he taught the original Yoga to the solar deity, Vivasvan, and then to Manu, the first of the Vedic kings, and then through a long lineage of teachers. Some regard Patanjali, which term refers to a serpent, as a manifestation of Ananta, the serpent on which Lord Vishnu reclines. Some regard Patanjali as a devotee of Sri Krishna.

The Gita addresses all the main topics of the Yoga Sutras including meditation, samadhi, Purusha and Prakriti, Self-realization, the Yogas of work, devotion, and knowledge, and with more detail or a greater explanation. In short, the *Yoga Sutras* is best understood in the greater context of the Bhagavad Gita.

The *Bhagavad Gita* is said to be the essence of the *Vedas* and *Upanishads* and is the core text on Vedanta. Most Vedantic traditions, whether dualistic non-dualistic look to the Gita as the prime text in their discussion of Vedanta. The Yoga of the *Bhagavad Gita* is a Yoga-Vedanta by its very nature and background.

Advaita Vedanta, starting with Adi Shankara, never criticizes Yoga in the context of the Yoga of the *Bhagavad Gita*, the teachings of Sri Krishna, on which Shankara wrote his own extensive commentary. All Vedantic gurus commonly write commentaries on the Gita, without which they are not considered to be authoritative.

This means that it is not a question of Advaita Vedanta criticizing the Yoga of the *Bhagavad Gita*, when Shankaracharya criticizes Yoga in his books like his commentary on the *Brahma Sutras*. He is questioning certain views of Samkhya-Yoga that posit an ultimate duality, not their teachings overall, which are largely the same. This difference does not extend to the Yoga of the *Bhagavad Gita* or Yoga as mentioned in the U*panishads* or in many other Vedantic texts. Nor does it apply to Shaivite or Shakta Yoga traditions that have Advaitic lines.

Different Systems of Traditional *Vedanta*

Besides Advaita or non-dualist Vedanta there are other schools of Vedanta. The school of Advaita Vedanta rooted in *Vedas* and *Upanishads* was renovated by Adi Shankara over fifteen hundred years ago, but the core teachings remain the same.

All Vedic schools of philosophy are based upon interpretations of the three prime Vedic texts, the Upanishads, *Bhagavad Gita*, and *Brahma Sutras*, as providing the essence of Vedic knowledge. Their founders produced detailed commentaries on these three prime texts to show the traditional authenticity of their views. There are slight differences or orientations between these Vedantic schools, though the main principles and teachings remain the same.

The *Visishtadvaita* or qualified Non-duality of Sri Vaishnava traditions as established by Ramanuja is widely followed in India, particularly in South India under the Sri Vaishnava line. Such modern Yoga gurus as Krishnamacharya derive from this tradition, which follows a more personal and devotional view of the Divine, including the use of images in worship (Murti Puja), the approach of Bhakti Yoga. It also honors Lakshmi along with Vishnu.

The *Dvaita* or dualistic tradition of Vedanta as established by Madhvacharya is similarly widely followed in India, particularly in the South, centered in Udupi, Karnataka and is likewise more devotional in nature.

Chaitanya Prabhu of Bengal and his tradition of *Achintya Bhedabheda* or indescribable difference and non-difference as the ultimate reality is another great tradition of devotion. ISKCON or the tradition of Srila Prabhupada follows this tradition as well as may others India, notably in Bengal. There is also the text of Narada's Bhakti *Yoga Sutras* which also emphasizes devotion (bhakti).

These forms of Vedanta do not accept the complete non-duality as the highest truth as in Advaita Vedanta. They aim at mergence into the deity through surrender and various devotional practices. Yet they also have very detailed, logical and indepth philosophies, sharing the main points of karma and rebirth, and the practices of Yoga and Bhakti, as well as the study of Vedantic texts, notably the *Bhagavad Gita.*

Bhagavan Ramana Maharshi in his *Upadesha Saram* notes the importance of Bhakti Yoga and the way of surrender, which he relates to Self-inquiry as well. Ramana never asked anyone to give up the devotional path they were following. **We should not reduce Vedanta to Advaita Vedanta and should honor the other Vedantic paths.** In addition, Ramana did teach the *Bhagavad Gita.* The same is true of Shankaracharya, whose devotional hymns to the Hindu deities remain the most widely chanted and sung devotional hymns throughout India, whether to Shiva, Vishnu, Durga, Tripura Sundari, Sarasvati, Ganesha, Rama, Krishna, or Ganga Devi.

The Hindu tradition identifies its deities in their highest status as Atman and Purusha, the Supreme Self, Parameshvara/Parameshvari, whether it is Shiva, Vishnu, Krishna, Rama, Ganesha, Hanuman, Kali, Durga, Tripura Sundari, Chhinamasta, in short, all the deity forms. The deities have various approaches or sadhanas to reach the Self. The deity itself is not the goal of worship except when we discover the unity of the Deity and our own inmost Self.

Sometimes people ask me as to how closely related are Dvaita and Advaita, I say that "the closest thing to one is two." If you can reduce everything to two, you can then integrate the two or duality into pure unity, like Shiva/Shakti, Radha/Krishna or SitaRam.

The other point to be remembered here is that such semantic differences of duality and non-duality in the teachings of great Vedic gurus are only outward. All these great teachers accept Samadhi as required to experience the ultimate truth of Self and the Divine, which is beyond speech and mind, and cannot be limited to name, form, or number.

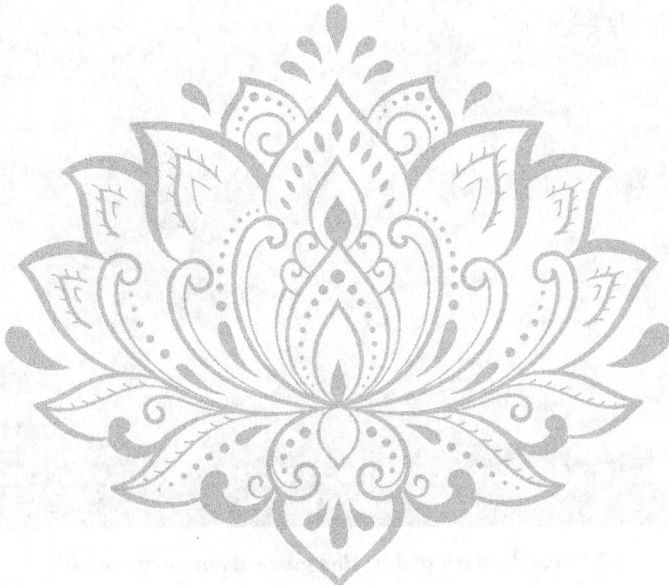

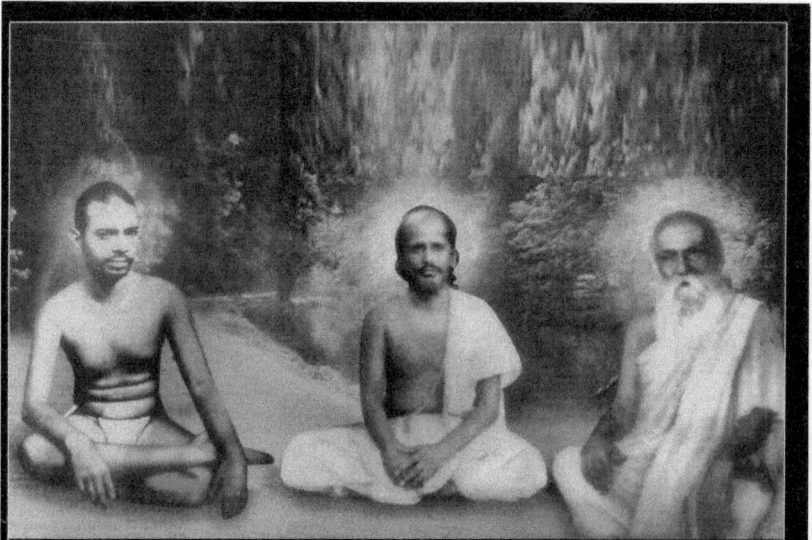

ಶ್ರೀ ರಮಣ ಮಹರ್ಷಿಗಳು. ಶ್ರೀ ವಾಸಿಷ್ಠ ಗಣಪತಿ ಮುನಿಗಳು. ಶ್ರೀ ಬ್ರಹ್ಮರ್ಷಿ ದೈವರಾತರು.

3 Great Modern Rishis: Bhagavan Ramana Maharshi,
Kavyakantha Ganapati Muni, Brahmarshi Daivarata

1.8

My Connection with Bhagavan Ramana Maharshi and Kavyakantha Ganapati Muni

Bhagavan Ramana Maharshi (1878-1950) is probably the most renowned and respected sage of modern India, the very embodiment of the highest Self-realization. He is known throughout the world as the master teacher of non-duality (Advaita). The picture of his illumined countenance has inspired millions, radiating with the highest wisdom and compassion, as if he were present before you.

Bhagavan experienced his full Self-realization when a youth of only sixteen years old after an extraordinary immediate inner transformation in awareness. He maintained that transcendent state of Self-awareness from that point on throughout his entire life. Everything he did from the most ordinary daily activity to all the profound teachings he gave reflected his transcendent state of consciousness beyond the mind and the outer world of duality.

To reach his state of Self-realization, though a mere youth he simply and directly with full concentration and dedication, meditated upon the inevitability of his own death. He carefully visualized the entire death process withdrawing from body, senses, prana, and mind, inquiring deeply on the deathless Self at the core of his being, searching for what within him did not die.

This powerful but short meditation of twenty minutes resulted in the permanent death of his ego and his mergence into the Supreme Self within the spiritual heart (hridaya). His inner focus was so complete that he never departed from that state of Self-realization afterwards. It became his natural state of being and way of life.

Ramana Maharshi is one of the greatest spiritual masters of all humanity, most of which had to labor longer and face more doubts and difficulties before reaching their full realization. Yet Ramana founded no religion, set forth no faith or belief, nor created any special order or institution in his name. He simply shared his wisdom and his presence with all who came to him, which gave them the opportunity to have a vision of their own Divine Self. His only possessions were his loin clothes. His residence was a humble ashram room that his disciples built and watched over for him. His awareness remained in the state of the Supreme Self and external affairs did not occupy his mind.

Ramana did instruct others, everyone who came for his darshan, regardless of age or background. Yet for him silence was the highest teaching, the silence of the Self in the spiritual heart. He had great disciples like Kavyakantha Ganapati Muni who saw in Ramana the presence of Skanda/Murugan, the fire-born son of Shiva, and Dakshinamurti, the youthful form of Shiva who taught the great elder Rishis by silence under a vast Banyan tree.

Such an exalted teacher as Bhagavan is extremely rare and should be honored as a guiding light for all humanity. His life and teaching is one of the most important spiritual events of twentieth century. He remains one of the main gurus for the entire world for centuries to come, spreading the transformative message of Self-inquiry, Self-knowledge and Self-realization for all, with clarity, compassion and grace, rooted in the profound Advaitic tradition of Vedanta, but as a living reality.

The Maharshi mainly stayed in silence (mauna) and only answered questions at certain times of the day. He directed students to their own practice of Self-inquiry, sometimes by a glance or in a few words. His was never any ordinary silence consisting of a mere absence of sound or lack of verbal expression. It was the profound inner silence and immutable stillness of the spiritual heart, reflecting an unwavering abidance in our true Self and Divine essence beyond all names, forms, words, and concepts. Ramana was fully present in his true nature, guiding others from within, even when externally he appeared inactive, with eyes closed. His presence remains accessible to devotees and disciples even today, notably at the Ramanashram in Tiruvannamalai, India but also anywhere we can call upon him with sincerity and aspiration to the highest.

The highest reality of Pure Consciousness transcends body, mind and external world, which are but its reflections and shadows. It is not the content of any idea, imagination or concept, known or unknown. It can only be approached through direct awareness and unmediated seeing, which is its very nature; just as light automatically dispels the darkness and no other special effort by it is required. To realize that we must merge everything we see into it as the inner essence and immutable being of all, infinite and eternal.

My Discovery of Bhagavan Ramana Maharshi and Advaita Vedanta

I have followed the teachings of Bhagavan Ramana for over fifty years now as an integral part of my life and sadhana. This began with discovering Ramana's teachings before I was twenty years of age, discovering the few books about him that were available in Denver, Colorado, the city where I lived at the base of the American Rocky Mountains.

Subsequently, I began meditating upon his profound teachings and his radiant picture that has entranced so many people as the ultimate expression of silence and peace. Ramana became my spiritual father, long before I first went to India. His presence was easy to experience within and around me, extending from the nearby mountains into my dreams and meditations, as a subtle but silent guidance.

This experience continued without break or forgetfulness as Ramana seemed to be present in all of nature, extending to the boundless space of the night sky as I had been an avid amateur astronomer with several telescopes. I did find a few friends who were interested in the Maharshi's teachings, but for them it proved to be transient or incidental, not a core experience as it was for me.

I visited the Ramanashram in India many times over several decades and wrote articles for its journal, the *Mountain Path*, which was kind enough to publish my young musings and contemplations. I had many powerful experiences at the Ramanashram, in Tiruvannamalai, Tamil Nadu in South India, where Ramana resided, and which holds his Samadhi. The monumental Arunachaleshvara temple towers over the city in which Bhagavan also stayed several years where the deities, Shiva, Devi, Ganesha, and Skanda/Murugan still reside and grant their darshan to those who have a sincere aspiration.

As someone who loves mountains, the sacred mountain of Arunachala, said to be the fire form or Agni Linga of Shiva Mahadev, which Ramana worshipped, particularly inspired me. I wandered along and up its slopes, meditating on the paths that Ramana walked on, saw sadhus wandering there, and climbed the top of the mountain several times, viewing the world from its Ramana inspired heights. The mountain is said to be a manifestation of the Sri Chakra, the cosmic world mountain and universal yantra. One felt it was on a higher Loka, not simply our human earth.

I visited the great Shiva and Devi temple many times where Ramana stayed when he was a youth at the Patala Linga, an underground chamber there, where he practiced the most extreme tapas in his perpetual state of Self-realized Samadhi. I felt a deep connection to the Devi and Divine Mother there whose presence I could feel at her temple shrine and communicate with her, exploring her connection with Ramana and Ganapati Muni, who also spent much time at the temple.

Ramana, Skanda, Shankara, Dakshinamurti

For me, Ramana expressed and explained the teachings of Advaita Vedanta and the great teacher Adi Shankara with clear, simple, and direct insights easy to understand and be motivated by. I studied the works of Shankara and Ramana at the same time, from Shankara's commentaries on the *Upanishads*, *Gita* and *Brahma Sutras*, to his special Advaitic works and his wonderful poems and stotras to all the Devatas and to the Supreme Atman.

I see Ramana as affirming and clarifying Shankara's teachings today, though teaching more through silence than philosophical discourse. Yet I perceived both Shankara, whose name is also a name of Shiva, and Ramana as forms of Shiva, not just as human persons. Both relate the Dakshinamurti form of Shiva, a youth of sixteen years of age sitting beneath the banyan tree teaching by silence all the elder Rishis sitting around him. Ramana is certainly the great guru of silence as a universal presence, not just the absence of any sound. Through that silence one can experience his deathless presence.

At the same time as I was studying Advaita Vedanta and Ramana's teachings, I was also studying the *Rigveda*, the oldest mantras of the ancient Rishis, which extol Agni, the sacred fire, as the first and foremost power of life, nature, the cosmos, and Yoga.

These Agni hymns reflect the same Advaitic realization as Ramana, notably Parashara Shakti's hymns that Kavyakantha Ganapati Muni has highlighted (Rigveda I.65-73), which speak of the search for Agni in the cavern of the heart.

During my meditations I came to recognize Ramana as Lord Skanda/Murugan, who is also widely worshipped in South India. Skanda/Murugan is Lord Shiva's son born of fire, an incarnation of the Agni of the Vedas, the destroyer of all ignorance, darkness, and impurity. Skanda and Dakshinamurti as youthful forms are closely related. Ramana holds that fiery power of tapas, the yogic Agni, which can remove us from all negative karmas and wrong thoughts. This inner fire (antaragni) is daunting at first in its penetrating power of purification, which burns us to the core, it takes us to the highest light if we are receptive and endure its transformative force.

At the Ramanashram I experienced the light of Ramana, which still powerfully illuminates the ashram and the entire sacred mountain, particularly during the autumn festival of Kartikeya, when sacred fires are lit in the temple and on the Arunachala Mountain in honor of Skanda's birth and hundreds of thousands of devotees have their pilgrimage, circumventing the mountain. This is the month of Kartika when the full Moon is in Kritika Nakshatra ruled by Vedic Agni, the Pleiades of western astronomy and astrology.

Over time I met with luminaries and senior devotees at the ashram, who shared their special insights and experiences of Ramana and their own Atman. Ramana did not create any formal monastic or disciple orders but left a lineage of inspired Yogis, Swamis and devotees of the highest order, which are now arising in every generation.

I was born in 1950, the same year of Bhagavan's Mahasamadhi and today am at an age older than he lived in his own life, but the inner contact with him remains as a constant guidance and support.

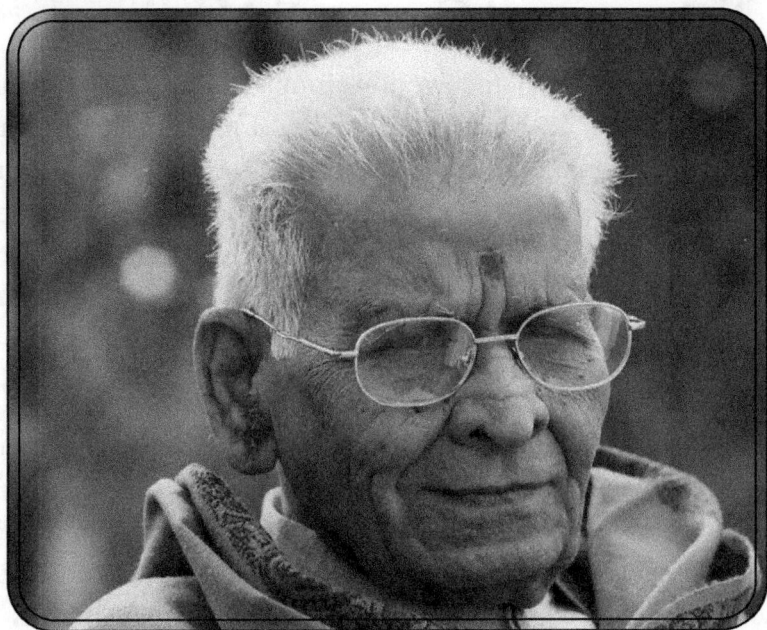

Close-up of K. Natesan

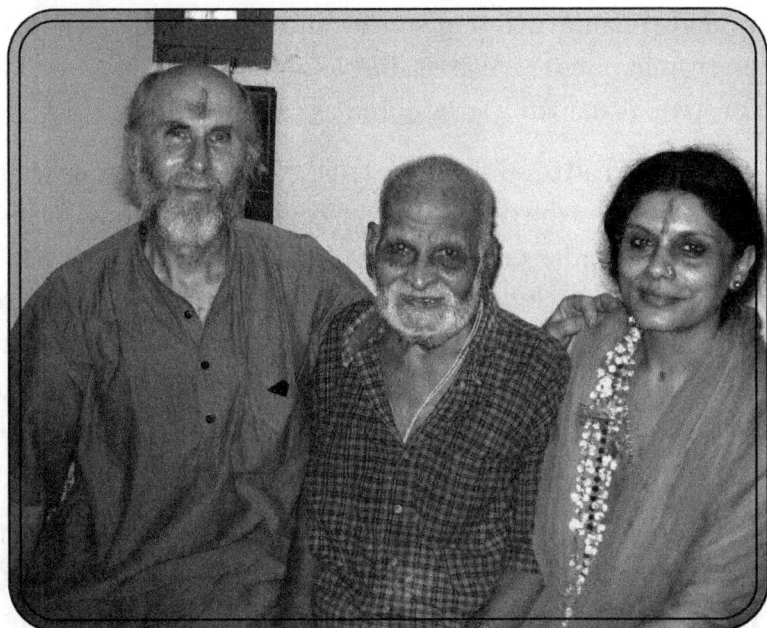

with K. Natesan

K. Natesan and Ganapati Muni

Most notably, I received an important and transformative guidance from Sri K. Natesan from when I met him in 1991 at the ashram where he resided in a special room to when he transcended this world in 2009 at the age of ninety-six, having been connected to Ramana since his childhood age of twelve years old. Natesan explained the teachings of Ramana to me in simple and direct terms and provided me a living link with Ramana and those who knew him in person and were with him on a daily basis.

Yet my connection with Natesan not only brought me more closely to Ramana but also connected me with Kavya Kantha Ganapati Muni, who was often regarded as the chief disciple of Ramana, one of his oldest disciples, and a veritable spiritual brother. Natesan provided a link with the Muni's profound Yoga teachings as well, which brought another level of teaching, mantra and sadhana into my life. The Muni was a Mahayogi and held all the secrets of Vedic, Tantric and Vedantic mantras, stotras, sutras and philosophies. While Ramana was honored as Skanda, the younger son of Shiva and Parvati born of Agni, Ganapati was honored as Ganesha, their elder son.

Natesan had carefully collected the Muni's numerous scattered Sanskrit works over the decades, often copying these down by his own hand, which he gathered from distant places like Gokarna. He gave me several of these hand copied volumes, many which then were not available in printed form or had never even published. Eventually Natesan was able to organize the publication of the Muni's collected Sanskrit works in twelve volumes, completing this monumental task just before his passing in 2009, not long after my last visit with him.

These volumes of the Muni's writings include the Sanskrit versions of Ramana's works like *Upadesha Saram* and Saddarshana and related commentaries by the Muni on Ramana's teachings, as well as the many other hymns, poems, chants, mantras, sutras and philosophical works of the Muni himself, extending to profound studies of the ancient Vedas, as the Muni was a prolific writer, poet, philosopher and guru on all levels of Sanskrit learning and mantric insights.

Indeed, Ganapati was the foremost Sanskrit writer and poet of modern times, and one of the greatest of all time. His monumental work *Uma Sahasram* consists of a thousand verses in praise of Uma/ Parvati in forty chapters, each of which is composed in a different classical Sanskrit meter including the most complex. Such a mastery of Sanskrit can only be compared with Kalidas or Shankara. Yet Ganapati was not just a poet, his *Uma Sahasram* overflows with all the secrets of Raja Yoga and the prime insights in the very mantric structure of the universe to the highest Lokas and the Supreme Brahman, including the very process of cosmic creation through Shiva and Shakti. Ganapati Muni also produced new Yoga Sutras and intricate and powerful mantras to the Goddess.

I have included the insights gained through my study of Ganapati Muni's presentation of Ramana's teachings in the commentary here on Ramana's *Upadesha Saram,* as the Muni's influence was behind the Sanskrit of the text. I have examined the Muni's teachings in my books on Shiva, Devi, Vedanta, Tantra, and the Vedas, which are only part of his vast learning, realization and yogic experiences which covered every aspect of the Vedic sciences of Yoga, Ayurveda, and Vedic astrology.

Understanding Ramana Maharshi and his teachings is not complete without honoring Ganapati, though their idioms are different. They represent the two sons of Shiva as Skanda and Ganesha, Skanda focusing on the direct knowledge of Self-realization and silence, and Ganesha having the wisdom of the universe on all levels, all deities and mantras. Both are part of a single manifestation and revival of the wisdom of the Rishis. It is futile to compare these two, though Ramana was the guru and Ganapati was the dedicated

79

disciple. You can see in this relationship between Ramana and Ganapati how a true guru does not make his disciples into imitations of himself, but draws out their deepest essence and Atma Shakti, for their own unique vision.

Sadguru Sivananda Murty

I received another powerful inner connection to the teachings of Bhagavan through Sadguru Sivananda Murty of Andhra Pradesh (Hyderabad and Vishakhapatnam/Bheemli). His own profound teachings emulated those of Ramana's revealing the Self in all with

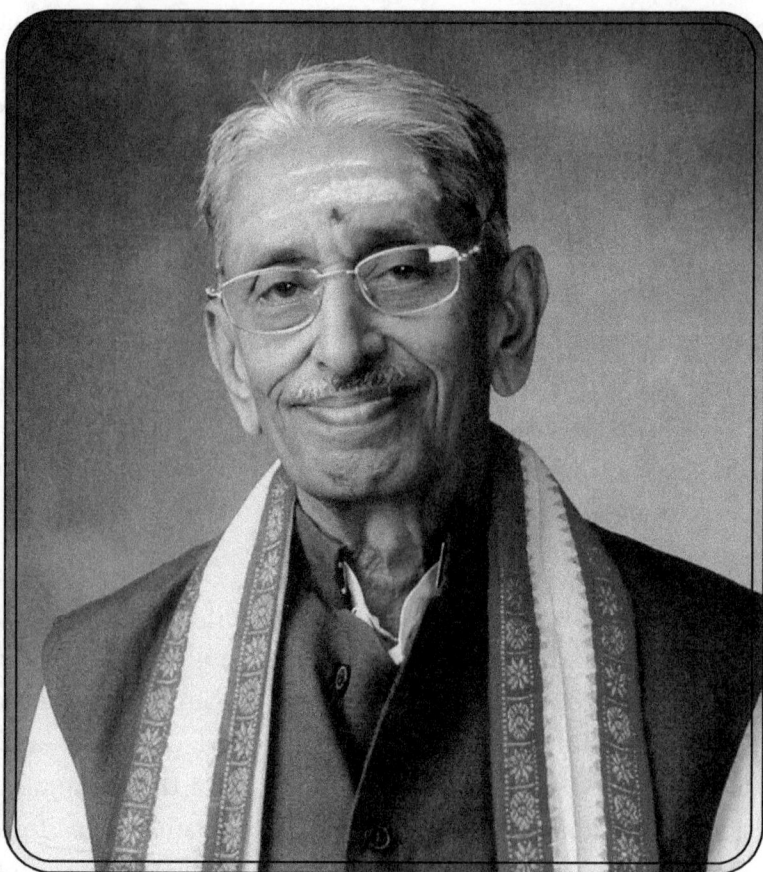

Sadguru Sivananda Murty

devotion to Shiva Mahadev. Sri Sivananda Murty was the head of the Shaiva Mahapeetham, an important South Indian Vedic Shaivite order and a great yogi and jnani, with extensive knowledge of Sanskrit, India and Telegu culture. He was connected to Trailanga Swami and Kashi (Varanasi) and to the Jageshwar Shiva temple in the Kumaon Himalayas which we also have visited many times and were deeply inspired by.

We were fortunate to have had the darshan of Sivananda Murty many times over twenty years in different locations, mainly at his Gurudham in Warangal, where his Samadhi is now located, and at his ashram near Vishakhapatnam (Bheemli). These meetings included various conferences in India and during his visit to the United States, extending up to his Mahasamadhi in 2015. Ramana's presence could always be sensed around him, as well as that of Shiva and Ganesha.

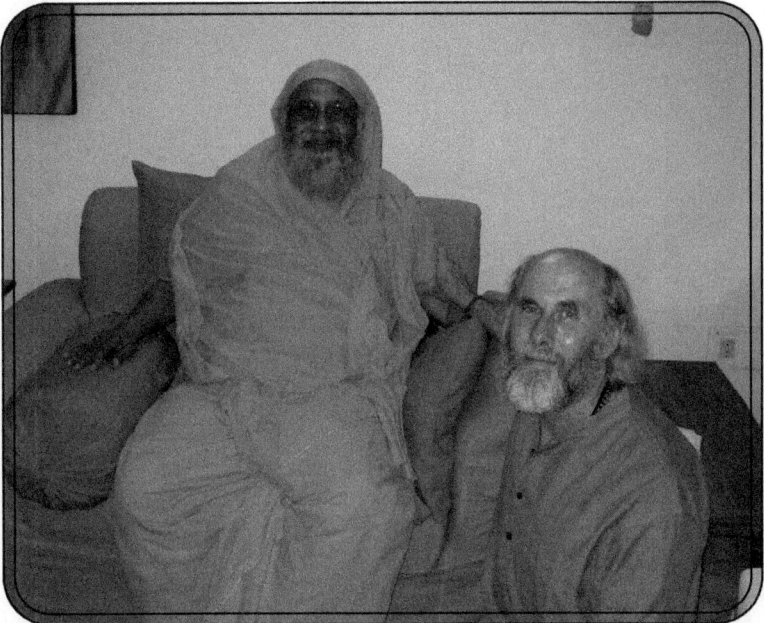

with Swami Dayananda Arsha Vidya

Sri Sivananda Murty shared the path of Self-knowledge and the Yoga practices that support it in a direct and lucid way, much like Ramana's teachings in *Upadesha Saram*. He was well honored and respected in South India, having been felicitated by the Shankaracharyas of both Kanchi and Sringeri, and well known to and respected by the Ramanashram. He guided us on all the deeper issues of sadhana. He sought the revival of India as the world guru according to its legacy of the Vedic Rishis and was well known to many leaders of the country. The Prime Minister Sri Narendra Modi called Sivananda Murty during his final days on this planet. Sivananda Murty also had a great understanding of the Puranas and all the many Lokas or realms of this vast universe of consciousness, which he could access through his own samadhi.

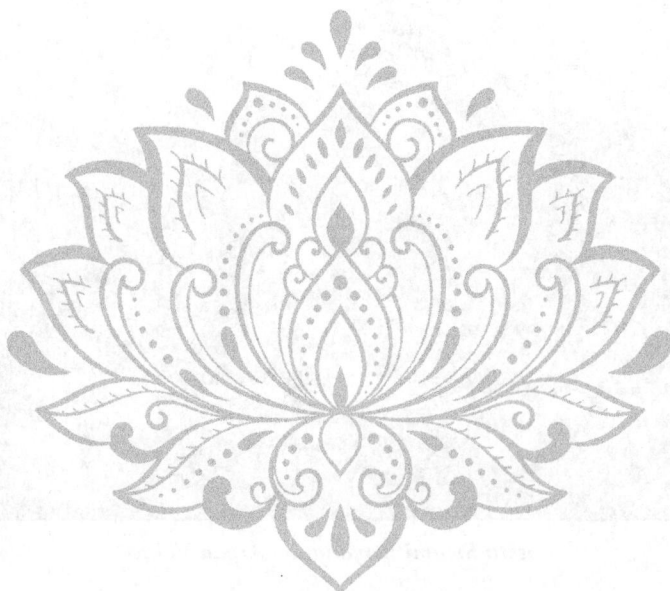

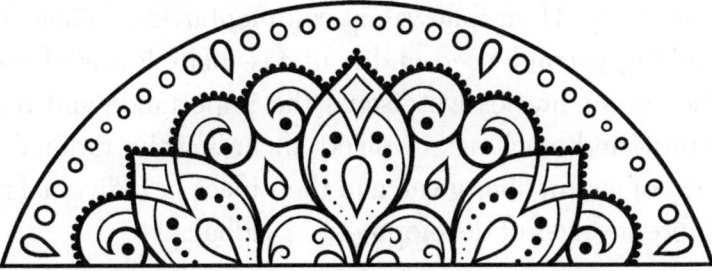

PART II
The Essence of Instruction in the Yoga of Knowledge

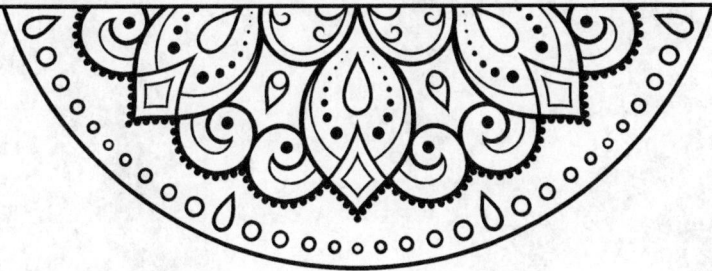

In the following section, we will present the teachings of Bhagavan Ramana Maharshi according to his profound Sanskrit text, *Upadesha Saram* which means the "Essence of Instruction". My presentation here provides the translation of the verses of which there are thirty. Then follows my commentaries on each verse, as the teaching is condensed and contains many levels of meaning. In these commentaries we discuss the importance and relevance of the profound teachings involved, including the rationale of the sequence of instructions given and their place in individual practice and different stages of development in sadhana.

It is possible to communicate this supreme truth of Non-duality to some degree by putting it into words; but we risk distorting it and making it into another mental formulation if we stop there. We can misinterpret a mere verbal or conceptual familiarity as a true comprehension of this very subtle and formless teaching, which the limited mind tends to do. Therefore, as we strive to understand the

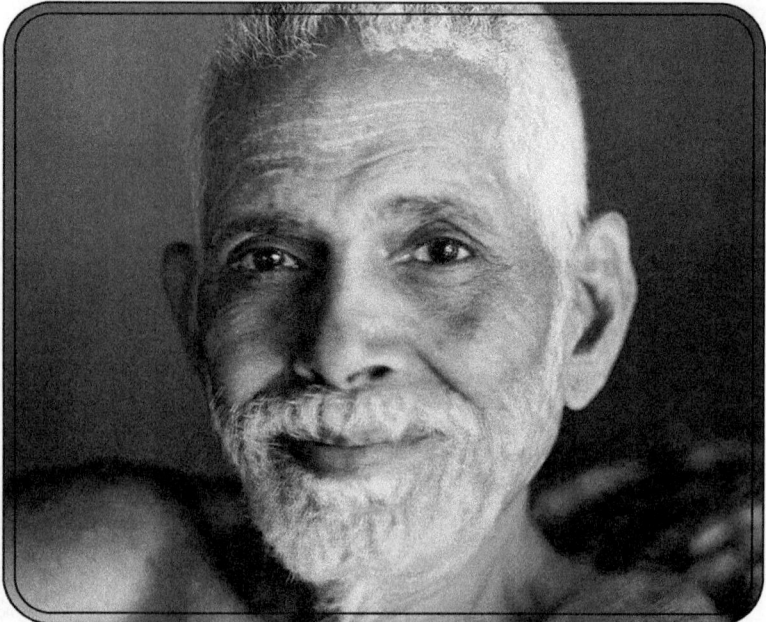

Close up of Ramana Maharshi

deep meaning of the words of these profound teachings, we should never forget the transcendent silence behind them, their inner meaning in consciousness.

Background of *Upadesha Saram*

The Maharshi composed few written teachings of his own. His native language was Tamil, which has many profound teachings, but he did create a few short texts in Sanskrit. These were composed with the support of Kavyakantha Ganapati Muni, who we have already noted a great Yogi and Sanskrit scholar of the highest order, and one of Ramana's earliest and most important disciples, like a brother to him, who gave him the very name Ramana and the title Maharshi or great Rishi. Kavyakantha and his disciples, notably Kapali Shastri, also provided the main commentaries on Ramana's various Sanskrit texts.

The Maharshi's teachings placed in such Sanskrit verses are concise, beautiful and poetic, reflecting the highest truth and deepest insights of the Rishis with clarity and simplicity. They are gems of wisdom to be contemplated upon throughout one's entire lifetime. Such works are like the new sutras of Self-realization for generations to come. *Upadesha Saram* is one of the most important of these core teachings in a mere thirty verses, though covering the topics, concerns and higher teachings that could be put into many volumes.

Upadesha Saram means "the essence of instruction." It succinctly explains the Vedantic approach to yoga and meditation according to Jnana Yoga, the Yoga of Knowledge, and how to reach Self-realization. Though short, it is regarded as one the most important works of Bhagavan. It is composed in one of the favorite Sanskrit meters of Ganapati Muni, will a lilting cadence full of Ananda.

This short text contains the secrets of many meditative and yogic practices and clearly outlines the way to Self-realization, making into it a crown jewel among the great Vedantic wisdom texts of all time. It should be widely studied, taught, and practiced with the utmost respect and the most assiduous application in inquiry, contemplation, and meditation. There is little comparable in modern times that so lucidly guides us to the highest realization in such a precise manner.

In this short teaching, the illustrious sage Bhagavan Ramana explains, stage by stage, the main yoga and meditation practices culminating in the practice of Self-inquiry leading to Self-realization. Its approach is simple yet systematic, thorough and comprehensive. He shows how aspirants can grow and mature from ritualistic practices, different methods of yoga and meditation into an in-depth Self-inquiry and finally into a full Self-realization.

The first half of *Upadesha Saram* explains the foundational practices of service (karma yoga), devotion (bhakti yoga), mantra and pranayama, which provide the sadhak with the discipline necessary to work with such deeper, direct-awareness teachings. Without purity and clarity or sattva guna in body and mind, this is impossible to achieve in any lasting manner. Mere intellect, however sharp, cannot enlighten us as it remains within the field of ignorance and partial knowledge, and the outer orientation of the mind.

Ramana always emphasized that aspirants requires a ripe mind (pakva citta) to authentically and realistically approach the practice of Self-inquiry. It is not something anyone can succeed in without wholehearted dedication, determined self-discipline and an enduring wish for liberation as one's primary concern in life.

Such preliminary practices as karma yoga, devotion and pranayama purify body and mind in order to bring this receptivity to the higher knowledge about. These cannot be neglected or dispensed with until this arduous purification of the mind is completed, which is never easy and is itself a rare and extraordinary accomplishment.

Yet if one stops at a preparatory stage of a yogic way of life and mind, one has created the foundation but not achieved the goal.

The second half of the text explains the yoga of knowledge (Jnana Yoga) in depth, along with its key approaches and methods, with profound insights and subtle practices that reflect the prime teachings of the *Upanishads* and Advaita Vedanta according to the ancient gurus. Ramana outlines the prime ways of knowledge such as the great Jnanis or realized sages have always emphasized but in his direct and decisive manner as a living experience that can inspire everyone from the level of the spiritual heart (hridaya).

That the supreme truth could be contained in a few verses is quite amazing. The text directs us to a powerful concentration on the teachings with the special mantric force of its verses. Each verse merits continuous and long-term contemplation. The verses reflect the prime axioms of Self-realization from which vast insights can be developed that transcend the mind.

The translation and commentary here are my own, which I have composed to bring out the deeper implications of the teaching, which are not easily discerned. Its aim is to help serious students access the original text and the guidance of the great guru behind it.

Toward a Deeper Understanding of Ramana's Teaching

Why would such another commentary on this illustrious teaching be needed, one might ask, when one can simply examine its concise yet comprehensive teaching? Though Ramana is well known, his teachings are not always deeply understood, and the path which he defines is like a high mountain path, not easy to follow or understand in its beauty and vastness.

Today, some teachers, particularly those following instant enlightenment approaches, have portrayed Ramana as rejecting all tradition – setting aside all books and all practices as unnecessary. They may present Ramana as teaching that anyone can gain Self-realization directly without any stages, whatever position in life or state of mind, not requiring preliminary purification practices, which they may portray as not only useless but also misleading diversions. They assume that by merely thinking they are the Self, without actually giving up the ego or removing their sense of bodily attachment, they can truly realize the Self, or teach it to others as a kind of quick Self-realization for all.

Such wishful and superficial approaches to Self-realization do not represent the tradition of Bhagavan Ramana Maharshi or Advaita Vedanta. They trivialize the extent of the tapas, sadhana and profound meditation that prepared these great masters to this very difficult goal – sharp as the edge of a razor as the *Upanishads* say. A goal as achieved only by one in many thousands who seriously pursue it, as the *Bhagavad Gita* states. *Upadesha Saram* provides a student with a clear view of the path and the necessary qualifications to follow it along its different stages that the individual sadhak must undergo. It ensures that the aspirant does not stop short with lesser goals. It directs the aspirant to Self-inquiry in an authentic manner, not as an assertion of the mere intellect or personality, but as a mergence into the unbounded light of Consciousness for which the mind must first be made receptive.

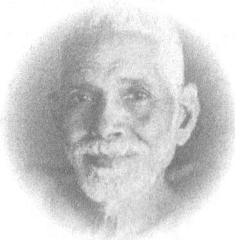

2.1

Background Qualification of Aspirants

Upadesha Saram begins with discussing the necessary background for aspirants who wish to follow the path of Self-realization. This involves the specific qualifications required for this advanced meditative inquiry, which very few will have the concentration for without any preliminary practices. One cannot climb a mountain if one does not have the right physical fitness. So too, one cannot ascend to the summit of Self-realization without the right state of mind, character and behavior.

Recognizing the Law of Karma

> *1. By the command of the Creator one gains the fruits of one's karma. Karma is not supreme. Karma by itself is inert.*

> *2. Karma makes us fall into the vast ocean of repeated action. Its fruit is transient and prevents us from achieving our supreme goal of liberation.*

To embark on the way of Self-realization, we must first recognize the law of karma, how it affects us, and what it entails in our life experience, so we can learn how to transcend our individual karmas and their compulsions. We must learn to understand our own karma and both its outer and inner implications, what is motivating us in life and where it will likely lead us according to our dominant thoughts, actions, and degree of inner awareness.

We must recognize that we create our own destiny through our actions in both this and previous lives, which carry us into the future by their momentum. To break this karmic inertia requires a powerful determination and dedication.

We must first assume "karmic responsibility" for our lives, acknowledging that what we do, and our resultant experiences are the result of our own desires, intentions, and actions, and cannot be blamed upon others or excused in any manner. We must free ourselves from the external karmic ties that pull our minds away from our inner practice. We must look beyond our karmic embodied self to our inner Self beyond karma.

The real pursuit of Self-realization is not merely another desire or interest of the mind, though some people may wrongly approach it that way. Nor is real sadhana and meditation another karma to perform or personal action. It should follow a dedicated aspiration to go beyond all ignorance and duality of the body and mind to our true immortal nature. It is a steadfast inner decision to move beyond all outer karmas.

Through the effects of our previous karmas, we fall into the cycle of rebirth and its resultant bondages and sorrows, whatever else we may achieve or gain in life. Until we face the implications of where our karmas are leading us, and become willing to change our actions and attitudes, thoughts, and emotions, we cannot move beyond the web of karma and its dualistic currents of gain and loss, happiness, and suffering.

Yet karma is not supreme or final. Karma does not exist by itself or proceed by its own power apart from who we are. Like the inertia created by the turning of a wheel, there must be some other power to set it in motion in the first place. There must be a higher force of intelligence in the universe through which karma overall works, as it is a mere force of reaction, not a true originating power.

Karma accrues owing to the will of the Creator or *Ishvara*, the ruling intelligence that governs this universe by the impartial law or dharma inherent in the very nature and movement of life which is all interconnected. This *Ishvara Shakti* or power of Ishvara supports the movement of karma, which has ordained it as a means of the *Jiva* or embodied Self's evolution in consciousness. We must respect the law of karma but also learn that by accessing that higher Divine will and intelligence, we can gain the guidance to move beyond it.

Recognizing that karma depends upon the Divine will and the operation of cosmic intelligence which directs the forces of nature, we cease to pursue the fruits of action for ourselves and look to the real power behind the universe to guide us from within, just as it guides the universe in all its processes. If we recognize the cosmic intelligence behind the movements of karma, we can appreciate the wisdom of how karmas proceed and transcend our karmic limitations.

We can let the universal divine force guide our lives and carry our burdens, so we can find lasting peace and happiness within, without worrying about our outer condition. We will no longer need to get caught in the cycle of karma by trying to impose our own personal will upon life, taking our outer actions and their accomplishment as our real purpose to the exclusion of our inner being.

Karma binds us to the world of impermanence and prevents us from contacting the lasting freedom of our eternal nature. Recognizing this spiritual fact, we gain detachment from outer actions, whose results are transient. This detachment is the basis of all yogic practices which require that we turn within. We can only turn within if we are not attached to the results of what is happening externally.

Whatever transient fruit we gain, whether wealth, enjoyment, or power, it must desert us in the end. This recognition of the impermanence of all life is the start of our deeper quest for the immutable. On gaining this detachment, we naturally let go of unnecessary actions and devote ourselves to our inner search for the inner Self.

The Necessity of Karma Yoga

3. *Action dedicated to the Divine, not done out of desire, is the means of purifying the mind and of facilitating liberation.*

Karma Yoga is the beginning of all true Yoga practices and the inner search for Self-realization. It requires giving up the idea that we are the doer and developing a deeper search to go beyond our ego and bodily identity, moving from our karmic activity to the essence of consciousness within us. As long as we think that Self-realization is something we can personally achieve by an activity of body or mind, or can put our name upon it, we are still caught in the ego.

The way out of the web of karma begins with Karma Yoga as detached and selfless service to the Divine within and around us, and to the guru or any higher dharmic cause. Selfless action purifies our minds (*citta-śodhakam*) and puts our lives in harmony with the universal consciousness. It is not action by itself that binds us but desire for its results for our own benefit, which we must learn to let go of.

Desireless action done with inner awareness is the foundation of all true spiritual practices and yogic methods. Such higher action should be free from selfish motivation. Yet Karma Yoga does not mean service work of any type or ritual done in a mechanical manner. It means pursuing excellence in all that we do as an offering to the

Divine, whether it is our outer duties or our inner Yoga practices. Karma Yoga rests upon an inner detachment and surrender, doing our best not for ourselves but for the good of all.

Karma Yoga has a special power to purify the mind down to a subconscious level and to disengage our attention from our personal desires and ego impulses. When we work with full dedication for a higher cause we forget ourselves and move within, letting nature do the work in harmony with the Divine intelligence behind it. This extends to our own Yoga and meditation practices, providing us the proper basis for a genuine sadhana. Action is performed by the instruments of body and mind, not by us personally. In our true nature we are not the doer but the witness of action that follows the laws of nature.

Ritual, Mantra, and Meditation: The Three Foundation Practices

4. The supreme duties of body, speech and mind are ritual, mantra, and meditation.

Rooted in Karma Yoga, we must reorient our faculties of body and mind, turning them into tools of meditation practice, not just instruments of enjoyment. Our individual nature and karmic conditioning compel us to act; and action to some degree is necessary to function in life and maintain ourselves in the world. We cannot exist even a second without mental or physical action, but we need not attach ourselves to it or regard it as our own. We must turn all that we do into an inner yogic quest for our true nature, with our outer actions performed as duty requires, not as desire compels.

Liberating action consists of yogic practices. These are threefold according to the three aspects of our nature as body (kaya), speech (vak) and mind (manas). For the body, puja, service or ritual worship is indicated; for speech, *japa* or mantra is the way for its purification; and for the mind, *chintana*, deep thought and meditation is the supreme prescription.

Our bodily duty is twofold as worship of the Divine and service to humanity and the whole of life. Our duties include dharmic values and a dharmic lifestyle, following the right life-style regimens as prescribed in the Yamas and Niyamas of Yoga and Ayurvedic life regimens. It may include the practice of yoga asanas to purify the body and reduce our sense of body consciousness.

The higher duty of speech is mantra, including the repetition of Divine names, prayers, and bija mantras. Such are single mantras like OM or HREEM, names like Namah Shivaya, or prayers and aspirations like *Gayatri Mantra*. The study and recitation of spiritual texts and Shastras is part of this, like the *Bhagavad Gita*, *Upanishads* or Vedantic texts. Such Mantra Yoga is essential for all higher meditation practices.

The higher duty of the mind is deep thought and introspection. This involves focused concentration, steady attention, profound contemplation, deep meditation, calm reflection, and Self-inquiry. It is not merely trying to blank the mind; it is developing the mind's higher insight like a mirror to understand the essence of reality within and around us. It includes the examination of the mind as taught in Yoga and Vedanta Shastras. Most importantly, it requires awakening our higher intelligence or *sattvic buddhi* through which we can develop discrimination and detachment, *viveka* and *vairagya*, the two main factors of all yoga and meditation practices.

The Twofold Karma Yoga

5. *Service to the world should be performed*
with our minds dedicated to the Divine.
One should worship the Divine, who takes
the form of the eight factors in the process
of universal creation.

Karma Yoga is twofold as selfless service (seva) for the benefit of all living beings and as devotional worship (puja) to the Divine in various forms like to the Divine Mother or Divine Father. Service to the world should take place with the thought that the world is a manifestation of the Divine and should include all of nature, not just human concerns.

True ritual worship, using Divine images and manifestations (*murti puja* in Hinduism), should acknowledge the Divine presence in the world, and pay obeisance to the Creator or Cosmic Ruling power (Ishvara) manifest as eight aspects of creation that make up the world of nature in all its beauty and wonder. *These eight factors are the mind, ego, nature and the five elements of earth, water, fire, air, and space, said to be the eight causal factors behind the universe, of which these compose the eight levels.*

These are reflected in different aspects of Hindu pujas and devotional worship and as part of Hindu temples. Without a recognition of the Divine dwelling within and around us in all of nature, any practice of service, prayer or ritual remains mechanical and ineffective, looking at the Divine only as an external entity.

Note that yoga asanas come under ritual as a form of bodily practice and should be done as a type of worship and performed as a sacred action. Artistic expression, whether music, dance, poetry, painting, or sculpture, can also be regarded as a ritual if it arises from an inner devotion. Any liberating ritual as part of Karma Yoga requires that we act with consciousness and surrender the fruits of our action to the Divine. Any action performed with inner awareness and surrender can become a ritual or sacred action. It is not just a matter of ceremony but requires an inner attitude of devotion.

Mantra Yoga

6. *Better than chanting mantras out loud is their soft muttering. Best is their mental repetition in meditation.*

Mantra Yoga relates to speech and is the next stage of practice after Karma Yoga, which deals with the body and our outer activities. Yet Mantra Yoga as speech has important implications relative to the mind as well. Our speech underlies and gives impetus to our thoughts. Besides verbal or vocal speech are deeper levels of speech at the levels of prana, mind, and consciousness that we should cultivate assiduously. Sound relates to the element of space and ultimately to the space of Consciousness (Chidakasha) and so can be used to even go beyond the mind. Speech is the root cosmic creative power and cannot just be limited to human speech.

Repetition of mantras takes three primary aspects:

1. Chanting the mantra out loud helps us imbibe the energy of the mantra and purifies the vocal organ, letting the vibration of the mantra reverberate throughout the body and mind, so that we feel it within us. It is the foundation of deeper mantra practice. This is the importance of chanting, kirtan, bhajans and stotras which sets up the mantric vibration within us.

2. Muttering softly or whispering of mantras internalizes the mantra and connects it with the breath, which it energizes as a force of awareness within us. A yet deeper stage of this practice is to repeat the mantra silently along with the breath. Most common is following the natural sounds of the breath as So'ham and Hamsa, "He am I" and "I am That." Yet any mantra can be given greater power if we chant it silently along with the breath. Various seed mantras can be allied with inhalation or exhalation to empower them.

3. Mental repetition of the mantra has the strongest transformative effect and can change the very nature of the mind, removing the negative qualitied of rajas and tamas (pride and ignorance) and creating the quality sattva as light and calm, the mind receptive a higher awareness.

The mantra can become our dominant thought and remove all negative thoughts memories and emotions however deeply seated. The mantra reverberates in the mind down to a subconscious level affecting every aspect of our awareness and prana in body and mind. The mantra naturally becomes a doorway to meditation, which it supports by providing the receptive foundation in the concentrated mind.

For those who cannot enter the state of meditation easily, which is most of us, such mantra preparation is very beneficial, if not essential. Mental repetition of the mantra can be done any time of the day or night. It can become the natural movement of our thoughts, transforming into a moment-by-moment awareness. Practicing mantras in these three stages is important, with emphasis on the third stage as meditation.

The Ramanashram, since Ramana's lifetime, holds programs of daily Vedic chanting. This chanting has the power to calm and purify the mind and generate an atmosphere suitable for meditation in the environment. The Maharshi recommended to his disciples the chanting of mantras like OM and various Divine names, particularly the name of Shiva or Arunachala Mountain (*OM Arunācala Śivāya Namaḥ!*), to increase the power of devotion. Silent meditation and Self-inquiry can easily proceed and endure after the mind is first harmonized through mantra.

Such mantra naturally becomes meditation and directs us into Self-inquiry. The Self is the origin and goal of the mantra. The mantra is our natural Self-vibratory force, which connects to that Supreme Self in a simple and direct manner. For this we must not only repeat the mantra but as the question: "Who is repeating the mantra." Mantra as primordial sound is not repeated merely by the speech or mind, but is rooted in our inner Self which is indicated by mantra starting with OM.

Concentration and Meditation

> *7. Like the flow of ghee in a steady stream,
> a simple and sustained stream of thought is
> better than that which is complex and broken.*

Meditation, of whatever type, requires steady concentration (dharana) or it becomes another transient mental activity subject to distraction. Such concentration should not be forced or mechanical or it will create conflict and division in the mind. It should follow a pure and unbroken current like a pouring stream of warm *ghee* (clarified butter), a natural flow. Mantras aid in this as a mantric flow of focused concentration in the mind. Yet formless meditation or Self-inquiry also require such a study flow, which transforms the flow of the mind.

True inner concentration is not a matter of trying to suppress the mind or forcefully stop it, which breed resistance and internal conflict. It means letting the mind flow inwardly returning to its source in the spiritual heart (hridaya). This can be achieved by cultivating a higher aspiration with dedication as in Bhakti Yoga. It requires developing a strong power of attention and Self-examination for the Yoga of knowledge.

In our current technological era of extensive outer media stimulation and distraction, such attention and introspection is lacking and often entirely lost. We follow outer stimuli blindly, not an inner aspiration with a vision. This distracted outer mindset is the enemy of meditation. The mind must be made one-pointed first before any real meditation or deep inquiry is possible.

Various yogic concentration exercises like *Trataka* (fixing the gaze), *Shambhavi mudra* (looking outwardly but holding our attention within), the use of yantras and mantras, or any other type of inner-directed awareness is helpful to develop such yogic concentration. We can hold our awareness on the breath, or on a chakra like the Third Eye, heart, navel, or root chakras. Wherever we concentrate the mind a deeper insight naturally comes to us and help us understand the nature of reality within us.

Ultimately it is our inner Self that is the most natural and easiest focus of concentration, as the mind arises from it as its source. Focus on the Self is the natural state of seeing and being. We must learn to access the natural flow of higher awareness from the mind back to its origin in the spiritual heart, which connects us to the entire universe. Such a flow happens naturally in deep sleep but in an unconscious manner. We need to develop the same inner flow in a conscious manner, leading our stream of awareness become a mighty river like the Ganga, creating its own path to the ocean of infinite Self-awareness.

Bhakti Yoga: The Yoga of Devotion

*8. From meditation on difference, one
proceeds to meditating on "He am I."
Meditation without a sense of difference is
regarded as the most purifying.*

To help the power of concentration develop, one begins with meditation on specific deity forms, such as images of deities like Shiva, Vishnu, or the Goddess (Devi), whichever serves as our Ishta Devata or chosen Divine form to connect to. This is the basis of Bhakti Yoga, the yoga of devotion, which usually starts with the worship of deity forms, though these are symbolic, and must be viewed at a cosmic level. Theis is the power of devotional concentration, which is the highest emotion.

At first one sees these deities as different from oneself, or as outside powers governing the processes of nature to which we are subject and must respect. Yet over time we develop an inner relationship, kinship, and intimacy with them, like worshipping the Divine as our true Father or Mother, the source of our being.

Then one comes to understand that the deities are aspects of one's own inmost Self, the Divine presence in one's own heart, mirrored in nature and reflected in our own minds. Such inner devotion culminates in the realization of So'ham, "He (the Self within the Deity) am I." There are many such mantras in Yoga and Vedanta, including the Mahavakyas of the *Upanishads* like Tattvamasi (Thou art that).

One comes to meditate upon the deity as one's true Self beyond the ego and all separate identity. This seeing of the Self in the deity is the real purifying power, not the particular form one uses to approach it, however useful that is as a vehicle. The form should be one that appeals to one's aspiration, which is why there are so many deity forms in the Hindu tradition, which teaches the doctrine of *Isha Devata*, or chosen deity: that we should be free to worship the Divine in any form that we wish or as formless, but ultimately as our own inmost Self.

Ramana worshipped Shiva with deep devotion, particularly as the Arunachala Mountain, regarded as Shiva's fire form, experiencing directly the form path of Bhakti Yoga but as part of the way of Self-inquiry. He also worshipped the Goddess and was in his childhood closely connected to Meenakshi, the Goddess form at the magnificent Madurai temple nearby where he lived.

Ramana's devotees saw in Ramana the form of Lord Skanda, the son of Shiva, Murugan in Tamil, one of the main deity forms of South India. They also saw him as Dakshinamurti, the youthful form of Shiva who taught the great Rishis by the power of silence alone. The fact is that the ultimate deity or Devata is the Self or Atman. We must learn to see that mirrored in ourselves and in all existence.

Formless Devotion

9. *From the absence of any mental state
comes abidance in the state of Being.
From the strength of that feeling comes
the highest devotion.*

Full devotional surrender takes us into a transcendent reality beyond any limited forms, ultimately to the Self within. The mind becomes empty of all thoughts and emotions and attains a state of pure unmodified devotion or mergence in the deity. One goes beyond any limited conception of the deity, and discovers a state of pure Being, the inner truth of the deity as the pure light of Consciousness and Bliss. From the strength of this inner awareness comes the

101

highest devotion, which is to see the Self in all beings and all beings in the Self, with the Self as the deity and the deity as the Self.

One should see everything and everyone as Shiva, Vishnu, the Goddess or whichever aspect of the Divine one most resonates with. This is the non-dual form of Bhakti. The Self that one discovers through this is not just our own individual Self but also the Divine Self of the entire universe, in which all the deities reside, and the supreme creative power. At this highest level, knowledge and devotion or Jnana and Bhakti are one. The highest knowledge is a feeling of pure unity. And the highest devotion is a recognition of unity all around us.

Abidance in the Heart, the Essence of All Yogas

10. When the mind attains complete composure in its abode within the heart, this is the essence of Karma, Bhakti, Yoga and Jnana.

The essence of all yogic practices consists of merging the mind (chitta, manas) into the spiritual heart (hridaya), the core of our being, which is its origin, place of rest and site of transcendence back to pure consciousness. Though different Yoga paths have different methods, approaches and attitudes, their goal is the same, which is to abide in the spiritual heart as one's true nature beyond all thought as the seat of the Divine within us.

This spiritual heart, hridaya, as Ramana explains is not the same as the physical heart or even the heart center of the subtle body (Anahata chakra), but the core of our being where the deity dwells within us behind all the chakras. Only there can one directly experience the supreme deity and the Self that is behind all. The inner

102

consciousness within the spiritual heart is immortal and continuous, with us in deep sleep, at birth and death and beyond.

Abiding in the spiritual heart is the basis of true Karma Yoga or action performed as an offering to the Divine in the heart, as all that we do while centered in the spiritual heart will be free of desire.

It is the basis of Bhakti Yoga or surrender to the Divine within, which must go to the deepest level of the heart for full communion and surrender.

It is the essence of Raja Yoga as silencing the mind through the eight limbs of Yoga practice culminating in Samadhi.

It is the power of Jnana Yoga or the knowledge of the Self, which requires the return to the heart to know our true nature. The spiritual heart holds the highest natural and spontaneous samadhi, through which bliss can enter into our entire life and all that we do.

After providing these foundation teachings, in the following verses of the text, the Maharshi focuses on how to abide in the spiritual heart, notably the two main methods of Yoga (meaning here control of prana) and Jnana (mind control and transcendence), as the spiritual heart (hridaya) is the source of both prana and mind, in which they merge.

The essence of his teachings is dwelling in the spiritual heart (hridaya) as the Self of all, which was the state of realization he entered into at the age of sixteen and which endured throughout his entire life. This search for our inmost Self is the Divine quest and our ultimate exploration and adventure in Self-awareness which takes us to the highest bliss.

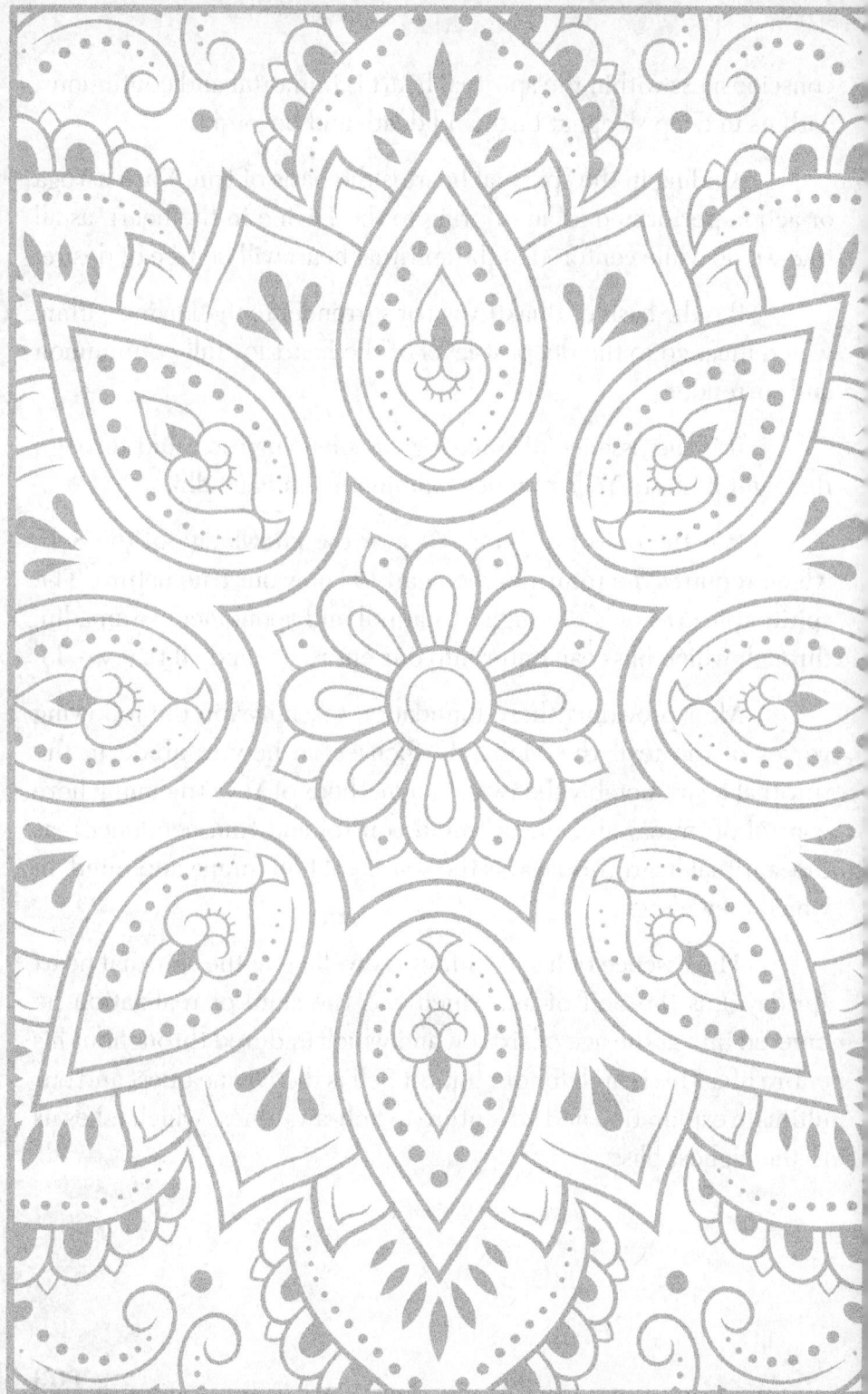

2.2
Breath Control and Mind Control

11. By controlling the breath, the mind comes to rest like a bird in a net. Breath control is a primary means to calm the mind.

By controlling the prana or vital energy through control of the breath one can also control the mind which itself moves by the energy of prana. Prana and mind are like the two wings of a bird as the complementary powers of action and knowledge (Kriya Shakti and Jnana Shakti). This insight is the basis of yogic teachings that emphasize pranayama in various techniques and with various mantras and forms of meditation.

Prana is the vital energy behind the mind, senses, and body. The breathing process holds that pranic energy in the physical body, enabling us to live, and energizes the body and mind overall. If that prana is not calm, centered, and unified, the mind wanders and becomes disturbed or dull, almost impossible to control.

Prana is mainly calmed through controlling, deepening, and calming the breath, which is its main instrument of operation in the body. Other methods to calm the prana also exist through control of the senses that disperse our prana outwardly, or developing will power which holds our prana within. Yet in all such pranic practices, these awareness of the breath remains important, making these into forms of meditation, without which these are merely exercises. Awareness of the breath detaches our consciousness from disturbed prana and mind.

105

We should note that only rare, advanced aspirants can control the mind directly, without needing preliminary pranayama practices to help them in doing so. For most Yoga practitioners, pranayama is necessary first to control the mind, helping to calm the agitated senses and vital urges that otherwise pull our minds outward. Through deepening the breath, particularly reaching a prolonged retention or the *kumbhaka* state, one naturally draws one's attention within, and the mind loses its pull towards the external world and turns within.

When the breath is calm, the mind is calm and naturally returns to its core awareness. That is why many Yoga paths teach special types of pranayama as their main support practice. Others aim at the awakening of a higher Prana within us, the Divine Prana beyond the body and mind, though devotion, concentration of aspiration.

Pranayama Practices

There are many helpful types of pranayama and breathing practices with various energies and effects, some requiring extensive efforts. In this regard the breath is like a muscle and only gains strength through regular exercise. Pranayama techniques are common in Hatha Yoga that emphasizes using the prana to control the mind. These are combined with mudras and kriyas and other yogic practices involving prana and the chakras. Kundalini Shakti itself is a pranic force.

To make the mind concentrated and one-pointed (ekagra chitta), which Yoga emphasizes, we must also make our prana and breath concentrated and one-pointed (ekagra prana). This requires balancing right and left nostril breathing, the solar or and lunar, pingala and ida nadis or *nadi shodhana*, to remove any pranic dualities that divide its energies.

It also requires balancing the five Pranas or Vayus within us (Prana, Apana, Samana, Vyana and Udana) and their different movements, Prana as internalizing, Apana as downward, Samana as balancing, Vyana as expanding, and Udana as ascending). This balanced and unitary prana facilitates the development of unity consciousness within us.

Yet perhaps the most simple and direct forms of pranayama, which is common in the Yoga of Knowledge, is simply observing or witnessing the breath from the state of the seer. Detachment from the breath allows us to move beyond its influence and naturally calms it. We can become connected through it to higher pranic sources beyond body and mind.

One views oneself as the witness of the breath, as different from it, which is outside of us, and withdraws from its disturbances, bringing the prana to a state of rest and peace rooted in the Self or Seer within. This is likened to catching a restless bird in a net. One can do this type of pranayama by a continual observation of the breath, which may be aided by the use of a mantra like So'ham or Hamsah.

Whatever you witness you become detached from and cannot be influenced by. Meditation on: "I do not breathe, only the body and lungs breathe. I am the pure awareness beyond body and mind. I have no breath and never die." When the flow in the channels of prana is turned within by the power of Self-awareness, the mind cannot move to the outside and therefore cannot get caught in the attractions and disturbances of external world. Removing the mind from external connections takes it to a natural internal state of calm awareness.

The Maharshi taught that if one is not in the company of a great yogi, which is quite rare, particularly today, pranayama is the best method to gain strength for one's practice of Self-inquiry. He was not against the practice of pranayama, as some have thought or even stated, but he did not make it the primary practice of his teaching but did recognize it as an important and often necessary aid. Those of us who do not have such exalted company or circumstances as a great guru or ashram to inspire us should not forget the efficacy of pranayama, particularly when we have restless minds and senses.

Pranayama purifies the body and the emotions and energizes the mind for meditation, granting a power for inner awareness. It helps us control the unruly senses that draw the mind outward, reducing the power of rajoguna by disconnecting ourselves from. Unified prana (ekagra prana) and unified mind (ekagra chitta) go together. Yet ultimately the Self is beyond both prana and mind, which are its two main instruments of expression as action and knowledge, not our real identity.

In addition, we should not overlook the many health benefits of pranayama, such as emphasized in Ayurveda, for increasing vitality, improving immunity, slowing down the aging process, increasing productivity and harmonizing body, senses and mind overall. The therapeutic value of pranayama is another subject and should be given its place in our lives. Yet for our quest of Self-realization, we must learn to merge the Prana into the Self within us that is its origin. We should not make pranayama an end-in-itself but use it as an aid for purification of the mind and meditation. Then it will help empower all that we do in our sadhana.

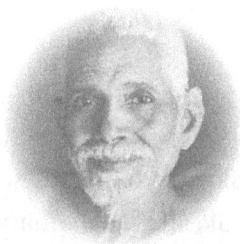

Meditating on the Shakti behind Mind and Prana

12. Mind and prana are endowed with knowledge and action. They are two branches whose root is a common power (Shakti).

The mind is the power of knowledge (Jnana Shakti) and prana is the power of action (Kriya Shakti). They are like the two wings of a bird without which the bird cannot fly or move. Knowledge directs us to action and action brings in knowledge, and so the two are interrelated. Both reflect the power of will, intention and motivation (samkalpa). Both mind and prana have a common power or Shakti behind them, which is ultimately the power of the Self (Atma Shakti).

One can control both mind and prana by going to their root energy, the power of consciousness (Chit-Shakti). In this regard one should meditate upon the power through which the breath occurs and from which the breath arises, the breath behind the breath, or inner prana behind the outer prana, as the Upanishads say. One should similarly meditate upon the power behind our thoughts, the energy of consciousness behind the mind and its capacity to know. This higher power of prana and of awareness is ultimately one. Life or Prana is a state of being consciousness. Awareness itself is a power of life and immortality.

You can merge your awareness into the pure energy, power or Shakti behind mind and prana, and see both mind and prana as its different functions. Prana and mind both arise from the power of consciousness and must eventually return to it. The Self holds the highest immortal prana that can never be diminished, as it is aligned with its eternal consciousness.

Our prana and its energization of the sense and motor organs allows our minds to express themselves. Our prana upholds the body, which is a tool of the mind. Yet our mind also has its own prana or vital energy, which allows it to expand or contract, ascend or descend, turn our or turn within. The mind is like light and prana like the lightning or energy it carries. Yet both are but reflections the Supreme Self that contains all light and energy in pure consciousness itself.

Ways to Control the Mind

13. Temporary mergence and complete dissolution are the two types of mind control. The mind that is merged will rise again. The dissolved mind is dead.

14. Through control of the prana, the mind is merged. From meditation on the One, the mind is dissolved.

15. The superior yogi has a dissolved mind. What further duty can he have, who abides in his own nature?

Pranayama and breath control suspends the mind from its outer thoughts and actions, allowing us to access higher states of consciousness and glimpse our true Self. But this is only temporary. Direct Self-knowledge in the form of "I am the One Self pervading all beings" dissolves the mind permanently as one no longer identifies with the mind or any of its thoughts.

Therefore, however useful a tool pranayama may be, without advancing from it to the state of direct mind control the aim of permanently dissolving the mind cannot be attained. One should use pranayama as a means to silence the mind and not stop short with it as the goal. One must progress from the calmed prana to the deeper awareness behind the mind. One must go beyond merging the mind into prana to the state of dissolving mind and prana into the Self.

The highest yogi goes beyond prana and mind by the power of singular meditation on the Self. The dissolved mind loses any movement of its own and functions like a mirror to reveal reality without distorting it by its own thoughts and desires. When we go beyond thought and action, we no longer have any duties to perform in the world or any karmic compulsions to drive us. We may act or not act as our inner nature and life circumstances allow. Abiding in our own nature we share the light of knowledge and bliss with all, beyond any external limitations or requirements.

Yet that the mind is dead does not mean that we cannot use the mind as an instrument of communication, or that we are physically or mentally impaired. It simply means that we no longer identify with the mind or consider it to be who we are, any more than we identify ourselves with our computer or cell phone. Such a realized guru can teach, write or travel, or remain silent and reside in a single place. Their inner Self-awareness is unchangeable and remain steady whatever is going on in the world around them.

The Supreme Pratyahara: Going Beyond all Objectivity

16. *The mind dissolved in the Self removes all sense of objectivity. The vision of pure consciousness is the vision of truth.*

The key to dissolving the mind exists in turning one's attention away from all external objects, no longer accepting anything seen as an object as real. This means regarding body, mind, ego and all of our thoughts as external to our real nature; which is indeed the fact. Whatever we observe in or through the mind is not our true inner nature or subjectivity but the mind's external vision, an object reflected in the mind.

Consciousness as Self-awareness can never be limited to any object, quality or condition that we can observe apart from ourselves. It is the immutable seer of all, not any object one sees. We must learn to negate all thoughts as different from our true nature, which is thought free awareness. All our thoughts and the mind itself are outside of us and do not belong to us or abide in any unchangeable state or condition within us. Recognizing this fact gives rise to the highest detachment; and then we no longer crave anything from the outer world. We come to regard body and mind as external vestures like our clothes and do not see them as constituting our enduring nature, real identity or true Self. When we are aware of this pure non-objectified Consciousness, we discover the ultimate truth of all existence.

This negation of thoughts is the neti-neti path of the Yoga of knowledge, in which we reject all thoughts as not who we truly are as I am not this and I am not that. Such thought negation is an extension of *pratyahara* or control of the outgoing mind and senses in yogic parlance. It is the culmination of the process of turning our awareness and prana within.

The control of the senses is the link between control of prana and control of the mind. The senses mediate between the mind (our thoughts and feelings) and prana (our vital urges). Having calmed the senses, we can go further and gain a complete control of the mind, by negating all our thoughts and emotions, realizing that they also are outside of us as well, like images seen in a mirror.

Ramana himself as a mere lad of sixteen practiced a total pratyahara or Yoga Nidra (yogi introversion) of the highest type, simulating the death experience and drawing all his prana and mind into the heart, which was the basis of his Self-realization. Without disidentification from sensory activity and external attachments, the practice of Self-inquiry is like gathering water in a vessel with holes in it. The water cannot stay.

More than rejecting the senses as external, one must reject all thought as foreign to one's true nature. Therefore, pratyahara should be practiced as the basis for meditation, extending it to the withdrawal of the mind itself. This pratyahara of the mind is the most important pratyahara practice, culminating in merging all of our faculties through mind into the spiritual heart.

Having explained how to control and dissolve the mind in a general way, the Maharshi now focuses on describing the specific methods of Self-inquiry to bring it about. When the mind has turned completely away from the external world, one can look directly into the nature of the consciousness behind the mind and contact the supreme light of Self-awareness. That is the prime path of the Yoga of Knowledge and Advaita Vedanta.

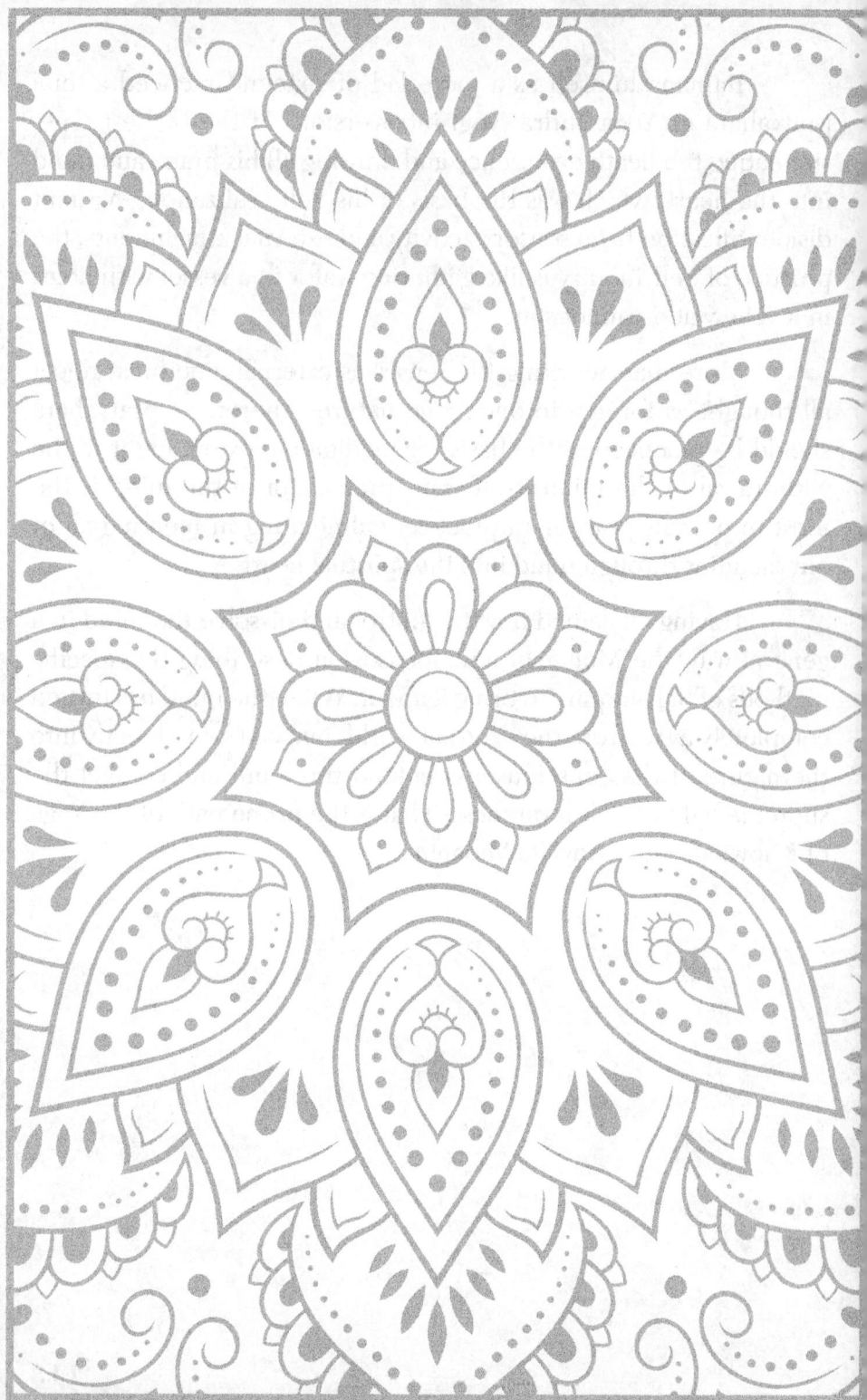

2.3
The Direct Path of Self-Inquiry

Questioning the Mind

17. What is the nature of the mind?
When one looks for the mind, it
disappears. This is the direct path.

To discover our immortal Self (Atman/Purusha), we must question our own minds to discover our true Self-nature beyond the mind. The mind is essentially an illusion-generating mechanism that blocks our inner perception of reality, as it is always looking outward. The mind is perpetually busy pursuing desires in the external world and creating its own imaginations of who we are and what we should do.

We are victims of our own minds that harass, if not terrorize us with an unending current of worries, fears, anxieties, uncertainties, and insecurities. The mind makes us run after endless speculations, hopes, and fantasies that prove at best to be ephemeral in their results, if we can achieve these at all. The mind is like a shadow or ghost that rules over us, a hypnosis under which we have fallen in a spiritual amnesia. Questioning the validity of the thought-based mind is essential to our ultimate truth, wellbeing. It liberates us from the mind's false ideas and their distortions in the world around us.

If we look deeply into the mind and how it functions, we find little enduring; mainly disturbed and distracted thoughts and transient opinions rooted in the subconscious and without any direct awareness behind them. The mind is largely engaged in wishful thinking and subverts the knowledge it gains and our education into an ego-based agenda of self-preservation and self-expansion in the outer world, which is the orientation of the collective mind as well.

Questioning the mind is one of the best ways to silence and master it. This means questioning our own thoughts of me and mine, and our ego identity as who we really are. In our inner consciousness are not the mind, but its witness, and can be quite content if we withdraw from the mind and its turbulent compulsions. We don't need the mind's collections of worries, gossip, fears or hopes to be happy and can rest content in our own nature as peace and bliss when the mind put to rest.

We must look deeply and inquire into what the mind is and what it consists of. We will then see that without the support of an external object or idea to depend upon, the mind, which always has an outer orientation and conditioning, disappears. *This questioning of the mind is the direct path to go beyond the mind.*

There is no mind as a real entity or power of its own. The mind cannot be located, fixed or defined. It is a cloud of memories, imaginations and expectations that have no place in direct light of awareness, which disperse it like the darkness before the rising sun.

If we search for the mind, we will not find it because the mind itself is a form of external seeking that is removed by Self-awareness. Apart from its stream of changing thoughts, the mind does not exist and disappears in the space of silent awareness. In the very seeking of the mind, the mind vanishes, as it turns the mind within, removing the outer orientation through which it functions. The mind is a shadow of the light of consciousness, a distraction to our enduring awareness. When we move into the light, the shadow vanishes as if it were never there.

When we look at life through an inner Self-awareness, we see that there is no mind, no known or unknown, no birth or death, no joy or sorrow, but only the play of consciousness, of which the myriad forms of life are but an illusory manifestation, a play of appearances. In the Self that is pure seeing there other reality. The mind's value is only as an instrument of dealing with the outer practical world, but it has no place in our inner transcendent reality that is Self-effulgent.

Self-Inquiry: Asking the Ultimate Question "*Who am I?*"

> ***18.*** *All mental activities are rooted in the I-thought. The mind is its thoughts. Know that the ego is the mind.*

> ***19.*** *Meditating "from where does this I come" the ego falls away. This is Self-inquiry.*

> ***20.*** *When the ego is destroyed, the pure I as the heart opens by itself as the supreme fullness of Being.*

The practice of Self-inquiry (Atma-vichara) involves tracing the I-thought back to its origin in the spiritual heart (hridaya). All our thoughts are based directly or indirectly upon the I-thought, the thought of self as "I am this" or "this is mine" or something that relates to me directly or indirectly. The ego is the basis of the mind, the very root of the mind, which is governed by desire and self-interest. When we cease our ego identifications, the mind must become silent.

Our thoughts are a composite of an *I* or subjective factor and an objective factor or *this*. We do not know ourselves directly but only according to an object, condition, or quality that we are temporarily identified with. This limits the I to an external appearance, starting with the physical body, projecting this bodily image on to the outside as our self-image in life. This scales down and limits our awareness, bringing in ignorance and compulsion, getting us caught in the wheel of karma and desire.

The way of the Yoga of knowledge is to negate the objective factor or ego and return to our inner Self beyond all external referents or outer identities. The ego is a reflected self or self-image that is the basis of the mind and keeps us trapped in the world of duality of self and other, subject and object, gain and loss, birth and death.

If we go back to the pure *I in itself*, the pure I am, the ego falls away as it is only a self-identification outwardly, not our true nature inwardly. Returning the mind and ego to the spiritual heart, one discovers Infinite Being as one's true and abiding nature beyond all death and sorrow. The ego or limited self is a fiction or misperception, confusing our inner being with some transient outer condition.

The true Self pervades all existence and is not limited to any type of body or mind. Knowing that is the most transformative realization that takes us beyond time and space and all limitations of awareness. This way of Self-Inquiry is Ramana's prime teaching and the essence of the Yoga of Knowledge, merging into the Atman or Self at the core of our being.

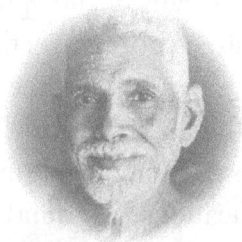

Meditation on the State of Deep Sleep

21. *This heart is known by the word "I" in our daily experience. Even when the ego is forgotten in deep sleep, it continues as our foundational being.*

An important experiential method of Self-inquiry is to trace the sense of self back to the awareness that persists in deep sleep when the mind is put to rest. We find this teaching explained in detail in the *Mandukya Upanishad* (and in my book *The Yoga of Consciousness*). It is the basis of the true practice of *Yoga Nidra* or yogic sleep, which consists of holding our Self-awareness during the entire sleep process, notably through deep sleep (sushupti). It consists of merging into our core awareness in the heart, in which deep sleep abides, which is behind and beyond the mind and senses and continues in the state of deep sleep, in which prana and awareness are renewed.

The background awareness in deep sleep is the true Self shrouded by the ignorance of waking and dream. The waking ego is an illusion arising from ignorance of our inner Self and identification with the waking body and outer world it lives in through the physically oriented mind. Once one has learned Self-inquiry in the waking state as a deeper wakefulness to our inner consciousness, one must carry it over into the dream and deep sleep states for it to become fully efficacious. This also means seeing that our waking life is but another type of dream and sleep, not truly real. Until the light of consciousness dispels the ignorance of the ego, our karmic dreams must continue in waking and sleep realms.

At the origin of all our mental activities is the Divine I, beyond the physical body of waking, the subtle body of dream, and the causal body of deep sleep. We must return to this original Self-awareness behind the veil of sleep and ignorance and break through it to realize our true nature. This requires that the state of sleep becomes an ongoing meditation, shutting off the mind but maintaining an inner witnessing awareness. Then our waking, dream and deep sleep will constitute a continual practice of Self-inquiry, revealing the unbounded nature of the Self beyond the body and mind.

Discrimination Between the Seer and the Seen

> **22.** *I am not the body, the senses, the prana, the intellect, or the ignorance behind them. I am Unitary Being. That which is dependent is non-being.*

An important Vedantic meditation method for Self-inquiry is to discriminate between the seer and the seen (*Drig-Drishya Viveka*), which is explained in detail in various Vedantic texts. This way of inner discernment should be practiced on all the levels of our experience. We must learn to differentiate our true Self, subjectivity, and sentience as apart from the various bodies (three shariras and five koshas), vehicles and instruments that depend upon it, and which we are falsely identified with.

This Vedantic discernment practice starts with discriminating between the physical body, which is a material form and instrument of action in the outer world, and our true Self of pure consciousness. The body consists of various organs, tissues, and material processes. It is dependent upon food, water, air and other external substances and energies. As such, it is very different than our Self-awareness and state of seeing, which is uniform, continuous, and independent. We learn to see that we are not the body, which is a product of the elements of nature and is composite, transient, and external to our inner awareness which is the pure light of awareness.

The inquiry then moves to discriminating the Self from the five cognitive senses (hearing, seeing, touch, taste, and smell), which are the instruments of outer knowledge based upon their contact with external objects. We are no more our eyes and ears than we are any other visual or audio instruments. Our cognitive senses are transient in their functions, being active at some times but forgotten at other times. These senses connect our body and mind, but our inner consciousness is their guide and can exist without them. The cognitive senses are material, objective, composite, dependent, and apart from our inner awareness. They are not our Self or inner identity but outer instruments that we use.

The inquiry then proceeds to prana, our vital energy that functions primarily through the breath. We are not the breath but the awareness that witnesses the breath. We have the power to observe our breathing process from a deeper awareness. This means we are not the vital force but the consciousness that upholds it from within. The prana sustains the various life processes in the body and mind, which depend upon its energy for their function, much like a force of electricity. But our inner nature and capacity to observe remains constant regardless of the fluctuations of prana that govern our outer activity and expression.

This meditative inquiry then takes us to the mind, specifically its intellectual or knowing power, the *buddhi* that allows us to determine what is true or false, real or illusory. We are not the intellect, which is an instrument of logic, perception, calculation, volition, and memory; just as we are not our computer, its memory bank, or its calculation capacities. We are the awareness through which these intellectual functions operate. Only when we surrender the mind inwardly to the silence of consciousness, can it reflect the light of true awareness. In that state we also go beyond any intellectual functions to a direct knowledge of immutable truth.

Finally, this path of discrimination leads us to questioning the ignorance or state of not-knowing which exists behind the body, senses, prana, and mind; that ignorance which abides in the state of deep sleep and shadows dream and waking as well. We learn to witness that primal state of avidya or not-knowing, the ignorance of our true Self. Behind that not-knowing is a deeper knowing, not as some outer form of knowledge but as an inner state of seeing. We are that true, self-luminous Self! Knowledge of the Self is the ultimate reality, while ignorance of it is a lack of inquiry.

The Self that our bodies, minds, senses, prana, and instruments depend upon is different from these outer formations. It abides in the spiritual heart and is responsible for all the activities and fluctuations of body, prana, senses, and mind. It provides the light and energy through which these can operate but exists in its own nature independently of them. These instruments are dependent upon that inner seer and knower, which is the true being responsible for their karmic states of becoming. Yet that inner knower is not limited to any of these instruments singly or all together. It is its own boundless knowledge which is Self-revealing.

We should learn to practice Self-inquiry not only relative to the mind but in our physical, sensory and pranic activities as well, turning our awareness inward in search of our true nature in all that we do. Self-inquiry is not just tracing the movement of thought into the spiritual heart but holding our entire life and existence at the core of our being. Every breath, thought, movement, or cognition can function as a means of Self-inquiry, if we inquire into its origin and background awareness.

Eternal Being as Pure Consciousness

23. *As the illuminator of Being,
how can Consciousness be different from
it? Consciousness exists as Being.
That consciousness exists as I.*

Another important ancient method of Self-inquiry is to recognize Consciousness, the pure I or pure subjectivity as the awareness of Being, one with all existence. This underlying I-am-that-I-am is I-am-all or Being is all. Once we have returned to the awareness of that Unitary Being we realize it as pure consciousness and our true Self. The nature of consciousness is pure light that illumines all things. That consciousness is the ground of Being itself, the foundation of all existence. Indeed, if Being exists it can only be conscious or Self-aware. An unconscious being is no reality at all.

Our true nature is the inner Knower, not the objects known or the instruments of knowledge like the mind and senses. As such, we exist beyond time and death, which apply only to our outer forms and functions, starting with the body. When we are fully present in our own inmost nature as pure Consciousness, we are one with all existence, manifest or unmanifest, known or unknown. We are Being itself, present everywhere and all times and places, pervading the whole of space. We can then see our true Self in all that we perceive, with no external object having any reality apart from us.

This inquiry into the Knowledge of Being (Sadvidya) is the basis of Ramana Maharshi's key teaching, *Saddarshana Vidya (Knowledge of the Vision of Being)*, which explains this approach in depth. Sadvidya is one of the key teachings of the *Upanishads* starting with the *Chhandogya*. Pure Being is the supreme reality. All lesser forms of being or becoming are but its appearances.

There are several ways to approach this science of Being. One such approach is to reduce the objects that we see into their foundational reality as forms of the five elements of earth, water, fire/light, air, and space. Then one should reduce the elements to space and space to the presence of Being that is universal.

Another such method at an individual level is to take all or our faculties of body, prana, senses, mind, and intelligence and reduce them to our inner Being and Self that is similarly universal. Whatever exists is part of the same being which is Self-existent and Self-aware.

That pure eternal Being is pure Consciousness and our true Self. In Vedantic knowledge Being and Consciousness are one. Being is inherently conscious and all pervasive. To realize that we must inquire into our own Being and discover it as one with the Being of all. The entire universe is our Self-Being and Self-Awareness. Seeing is Being. Whatever you truly see with the vision of Self-knowledge, you are that. Every form of being that you see is one with your own Being that is the being of all.

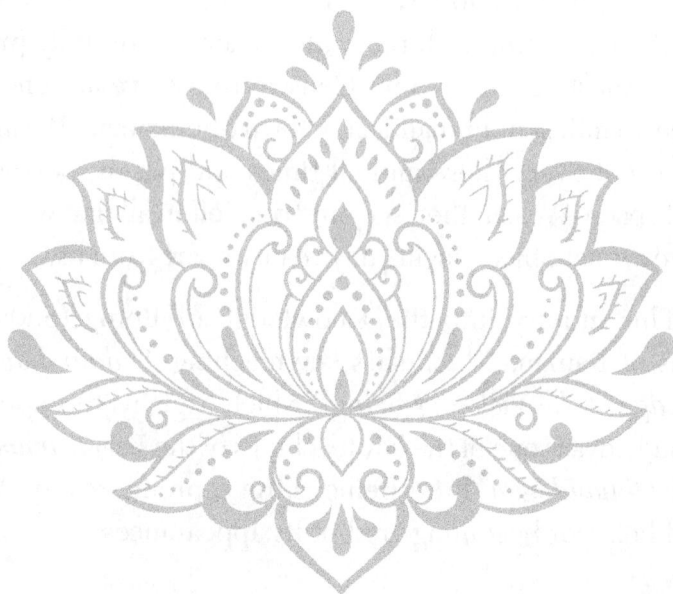

Merging God (Ishvara) and the Soul (Jivatman) into the Supreme Self (Paramatman)

24. *God (Ishvara) and the soul (Jiva) are differentiated only by their vestures. Their Self-nature as pure being is the supreme reality.*

25. *By eliminating the differing vestures in the perception of the Self-nature, the vision of the Divine takes the form of the Self within.*

Ishvara and *Jiva*, the Cosmic Creator, and the embodied creature, are the two ultimate factors behind the universe which constitutes their field of action. Yet these two differ only by their outer vestures, the bodies and minds that they assume. Inwardly they are one.

Ishvara as the ruling cosmic intelligence has an all-powerful mind and prana, not limited to a body or birth and death. His mind is the cosmic mind and supreme intelligence called *Mahat Tattva* in yogic thought, which holds the highest knowledge inherent within it, of which our human intelligence is but a mere spark.

Ishvara's intelligence never falls under ignorance or avidya. It is composed of pure sattva, the quality of light and intelligence, Ishvara through his Shakti rules over all the processes in the universe, starting with the law of karma and the dharmic principles governing all life.

Ishvara's prana is the immortal Cosmic Prana that creates all the worlds and upholds the various dimensions of the universe, of which our human life is but a small aspect. His prana is never subject to death or sorrow. Ishvara is the original guru of Yoga as mentioned in the *Yoga Sutras*. It is the cosmic Self-awareness behind the universe that links us to the Supreme Self-awareness beyond all manifestation. The universe is the Self-manifestation of Ishvara as the Self-awareness behind the universe.

The Jivatman as the reincarnating individual being has a limited mind and limited prana along with an ego in each of its lives. Our minds are limited by the ego or bodily identity, with our intelligence also limited, caught in the shadow of the external world of Maya. Our senses are limited and superficial in their perception, not revealing the inner truth but only the outer form. Our minds rest upon the physical body that has many limitations in size, movement and energy, as well as a short term of life. Our will power and vitality are limited as well, reflecting our creaturely desires and compulsions, and the entropy our karmas.

Yet the common Self-nature between Ishvara and the Jiva unites them in the supreme reality of Brahman, the Transcendent Absolute beyond all names and forms, bodies and minds, even beyond the Cosmic Mind and Cosmic Prana. The way to unite Ishvara and the Jivatman is to look beyond their outer vestures and manifest forms and recognize the common Consciousness behind them.

The Being within the Creator or what could be called God (Ishvara) and the Being within the individual soul (Jivatman) is the same Unbounded and Immutable Being. One can only truly know God or the Divine as the Self, not as an object, idea, or any separate entity. Any other knowledge of God or the Creator is indirect and not real, just an emotion or mental concept.

Yet to know that Supreme Divine one must remove the veil of one's "individual" human personality and mind to reveal the all-pervading Self that is our true nature and the nature of the entire universe. This requires a radical change of awareness through the process of Self-inquiry, uncovering the same Self and Being within all. God and the reincarnating soul are one in the Supreme Self.

Abidance in the Self

26. The state of the Self is the seeing of the Self. From the non-dual nature of the Self arises abidance in the Self.

Meditating on the unity of being and seeing is another important approach to realize the Self. Being is always Self-luminous, which means it is the seer of all. Being is Seeing and Seeing is Being. There is no particular method required do this because the Self is simply what it is, which is the light of being and seeing as the same power. You are what you are. You cannot be an other, an object or an action, to yourself. Your being is intrinsic.

To see and be aware is to be and to be all. To see the Self is to be the Self. To be the Self is to see the Self. The Self is of the nature of light and is always Self-revealing as long as we are not seeking out any external objects or desires.

The Self is only one, beyond all duality, apart from all name, form, number, time, space and karma. It is the natural state of awareness within the core of our being, the spiritual heart (hridaya). To know the Self, we must be who we are in the core of our being, apart from all changing outer identities or involvements.

To dwell in the Self, we must let go of all that is not-Self, which includes anything we have been identified with, and all that we can perceive on the outside through the mind. We are pure identity that is all pervasive and one with all, not any limited identity as opposed to another. Then unbounded Self-effulgence becomes our abiding reality of pure Ananda, peace and bliss absolute.

Beyond the Known and the Unknown

27. *Consciousness devoid of knowing and not knowing is the real knowledge. What else is there to know?*

Another transformative method of the Yoga of Knowledge to realize the Self is to meditate on "What is knowledge?" Meditation upon what constitutes real knowledge reveals the nature of Eternal Reality. Such direct knowledge is very different from information of various types. What is the nature of outer knowledge that is transient and superficial and what is true inner knowledge which is direct awareness?

What we call knowledge is mere information that has little enduring value and cannot enable us to understand who we truly are or what is the real meaning of our lives or the universe. Information is just knowledge of the shadows of the outer world in the dance of time and space, transient appearances only, not the immortal inner Being.

Our ordinary knowledge about external reality is defined by name, form, or number, not an inward cognition of the nature of eternal reality. Such outer knowledge is bound by ignorance and sorrow, trapped in changing boundaries and uncertain appearances. It may have practical value in our physical lives for dealing with the material world, but it has no existential reality. It can help us function in the outer world relative to our personal and social needs, but cannot tell us what is beyond it, or who we really are apart from our outer form and expression.

There is a higher form knowledge than all that we can possibly know with our minds, our senses, and scientific instruments. The highest knowledge is Self-knowledge, knowing our true nature in pure consciousness beyond all name, form or number. This highest knowledge is devoid of any object to be known or any instrument to know it with. It is devoid of any outer knower who owns or collects it. It is self-luminous, self-aware wisdom without any thought or modification. It is not knowledge about anything but knowledge in itself as intrinsic Self-knowing.

The highest knowing requires going beyond all that we call knowledge even in science. This is not a mere theoretical leap into a blank state of mind but a revolution at the core of consciousness. This knowledge is the state of unity consciousness that sees the same Self in all beings, pervading the entire universe. It is an inherent and intrinsic knowing, not a form of knowledge gained or described, explaining something particular or form-based.

At the highest level, there is nothing to know and no one who could possibly know it, no real separate mind and no outer object apart from us. We could call this higher knowledge the "supreme unknowing", in which all else is forgotten, which abides far beyond all the appearances of the world, actual or imaginary. There is only the inherent knowledge of pure existence that requires no instrument, no agency, no means of knowledge, and no effort to know. At the highest level, there is no effort to be aware, as awareness is the nature of all that is, a spontaneous illumination, a Self-effulgence beyond any need to know.

Bliss (Ananda) Absolute

28. *What is the Self-nature? In the perception of the Self is the immutable, unborn, consciousness bliss absolute.*

29. *He who here attains the supreme bliss beyond bondage and release lives a Divine life.*

Self-inquiry means is search out the ultimate source of bliss or true happiness within us. We are all searching for enduring happiness, which is our main quest in life. No one wants to be unhappy because happiness (Ananda) is our true nature. The problem is that we are seeking for happiness outwardly, but happiness that exists externally can never belong to us in any lasting manner. Any outward source of happiness, whether in property, wealth, pleasure, relationship, or recognition remains outside of us and cannot fulfill our inner search for abiding bliss.

Ultimate happiness dwells only in the Self, not in any external object or condition of mental or sensory enjoyment. Indeed, what happiness can we have apart from our own awareness which experiences it? If we are not there, what happiness can we have? This means that true happiness is found only in our inner consciousness, not in any material acquisition or achievement. Attaining happiness that is our true nature must be our true search for lasting happiness to be possible.

This bliss (ananda) of the Self is the basis of the peace and happiness that we experience in the state of deep sleep, which renews our wellbeing every day. It extends to yogic samadhis that arise in our sadhana, and ultimately to the highest samadhi of Self-realization. If we cannot find this inner happiness, the pursuit of outer happiness must lead to eventual loss and sorrow. If we have this inner contentment, then any outer pleasures will have no appeal for us and not be able to attract or influence our minds. Our inner nature is happiness. We only need reclaim that by looking within. It need not be borrowed from elsewhere or pursued on the outside as an object apart from us.

The individual Jiva becomes the Supreme Self (Paramatman) by going back to its true nature at the core of its being beyond joy and sorrow or any concepts of the mind. This is the supreme goal of practice that is beyond all goals and all practices, returning to the Divine source. To reach it is the highest bliss and peace. Yet in the end all meditation practices fall away, as we return to our source in pure consciousness, in which they are no longer necessary. The Self-realized individual lets go of these like leaving behind the boat one uses to cross the water once one has reached the other shore. This supreme bliss or *Paramananda* is the origin, support, and end of everything. Beyond that nothing needs to be said or accomplish.

The inquiry into happiness and Ananda is one of the main ways of knowledge in the *Upanishads*, extending throughout Yoga and Vedanta. Going beyond sorrow and discovering bliss is the prime motivation of human life. Yet only that *Atmananda* or Bliss of the Self can grant that to us, which is the highest and most natural Samadhi.

Summary of Ramana Maharshi's Teaching

30. One's own awareness free of the ego—this is the great austerity and the Word of Ramana.

This pure awareness beyond the separate self is the highest knowledge and deepest wisdom. It is not conceptual, verbal, quantitative or mental in nature or dependent upon anything on the outside It is like a great fire (Mahan Agni) that burns away all

131

thoughts and desires, removing all dualities and contraries. It is *tapas*, an intense concentration like a burning fire that purifies all else. The Maharshi manifested this unbroken Self-awareness in his daily way of life rooted in the ultimate simplicity and the highest truth. Ramana did not simply talk about Self-realization or teach it as a theory, imagination or emotion. He lived it at every moment, with his awareness naturally abiding beyond the ego and body consciousness.

This teaching beyond the ego is Ramana's Divine Word and mantra, not simply a mental utterance or verbal formulation. It arose from the Divine I am in the spiritual heart (hridaya), not a product of human thought or speculation.

This fire of tapas is why Ramana was equated with Shiva's son Lord Skanda (Murugan) who was born of fire, and of the Arunachala form of Shiva himself, which is Shiva's fire form. Ramana was a manifestation of that supreme Agni from which all the Vedas arose, and which gives light to all. That inner Agni in the cave of the heart is the abode of the Supreme Self which the inner journey of Self-inquiry leads us to.

It is not difficult to read such profound teachings of Vedanta and to understand these logically or at a theoretical level. One can use them to create a mental or emotional inspiration. Yet their full true realization requires a tremendous, steadily focused meditation practice. This is not merely following a technique, or moving the body, prana, or mind in a certain manner, but constantly engaging one's attention within regardless of the ups and downs of the outer world. It is to be immersed in continued moment-by-moment awareness, introspection, and Self-inquiry.

To reach that focused Self-awareness we must dedicate ourselves to it as the primary endeavor in all that we do, consider, or aspire to. Our lives should be an enduring movement in introspection,

Self-observation, and Self-inquiry – looking ever more deeply within ourselves and behind the forces of nature to the Self of all.

The Maharshi offers this supreme teaching to us as his blessing, as his expression of the Divine Word, the vibratory essence of the cosmic reality indicated by OM. Ramana embodied this supreme teaching in the human world and sustains it in the Cosmic Mind. We can approach this inner teaching with his guidance and his grace if we are receptive to its power and his compassion.

As our true Self and inner guru, Bhagavan Ramana Maharshi abides within us, directing us from within beyond the mind and all Samsara. We can become one with his inner Consciousness whenever we are willing to let go of our ego, mind, and our bodily identity – and dare to be free in the infinite space of Pure Being. In that all name, form and person merge in the Supreme Self. In this way the Maharshi returns us to our spiritual heart in which we are one with all.

If we study this teaching of a mere thirty verses and put it into practice in our daily lives, as our mantra, meditation, and Self-inquiry, we can discover that Self of all as our true, immortal, and infinite reality.

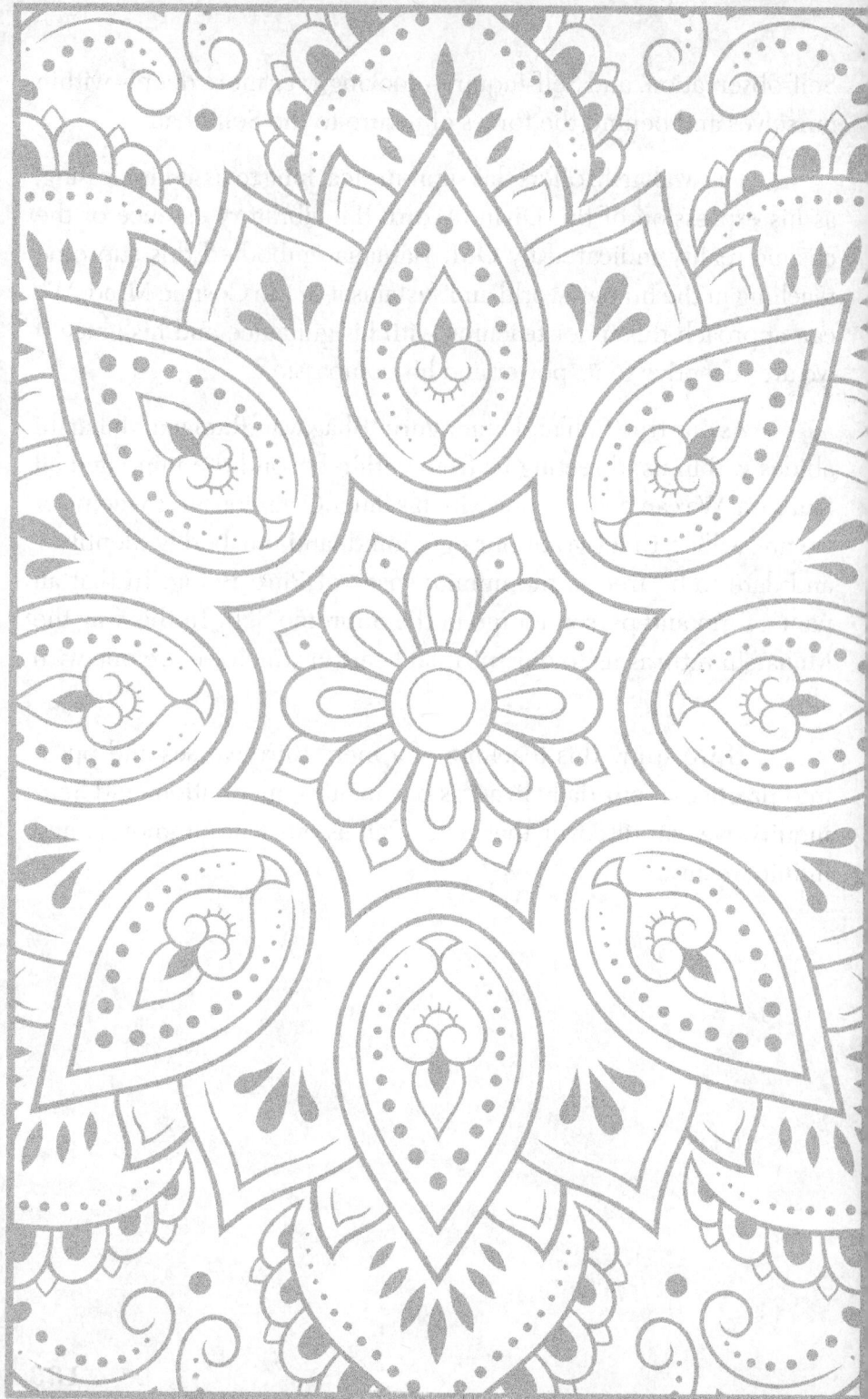

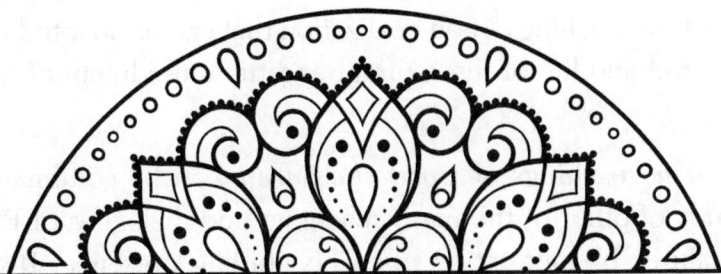

PART III
Keys to the Application of the Non-dual Teaching

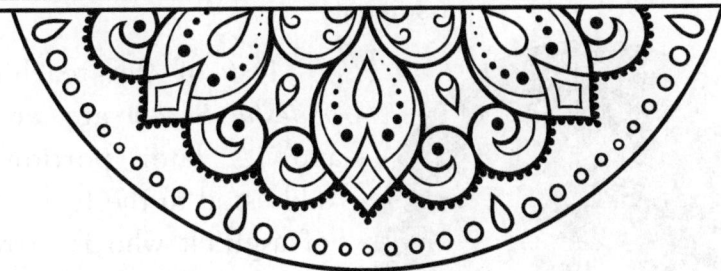

This in-depth approach to Self-realization summarizes both the preliminary and advanced teachings of the Yoga of Knowledge (Jnana Yoga), centered on Self-inquiry (Atma Vichara), and guiding us in its application and unfoldment. Its approach constitutes a complete yet practical teaching of Self-realization that can be adapted relative to the level and life of the aspirant and the unfoldment of the Self within.

The teachings of *Upadesha Saram* can be combined with the study of other of the many teachings and dialogues of Ramana Maharshi or by meditating upon his abiding presence. It can be learned along with the teachings of great masters of Advaita Vedanta of ancient and modern times, like Yajnavalkya in the *Upanishads*, Krishna in the *Gita*, Adi Shankara, or the Swamis and Shankaracharyas today. It can be integrated into yogic practices to purify the body, prana, senses, and mind performed to develop the way forward to reach it.

After examining this magnificent and profound teaching, which elucidates the supreme truth of Self-realization, the question then arises for each individual aspirant as to how to apply the teaching in the best possible manner for oneself, one's level of awareness and different life circumstances, which can be quite variable or even contrary to these higher truths, presenting many obstructions to pursuing it.

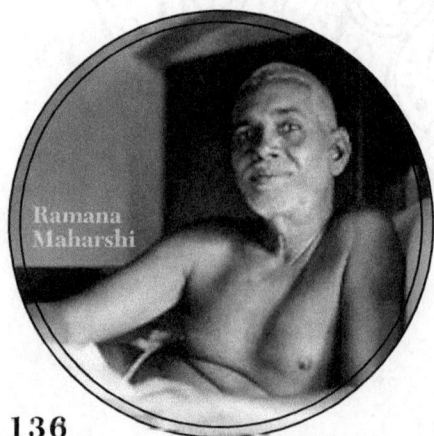

Ramana
Maharshi

Most of the teaching in *Upadesha Saram* are advanced and its later portions are addressed to the highest level of aspirant who is extremely rare to find, particularly in our turbulent world today. Even its preliminary instructions are hard to put into an enduring practice, however clear the ideas and insights might appear to be at an intellectual level. The subtlety and sharpness of intelligence required for Self-inquiry is outside of our educational system on all levels, even our so-called higher education.

Our current materialistic social order and outward looking information technology adds additional challenges to the path of Self-inquiry, which is always daunting. The intellectual ego itself can be the greatest obstruction, thinking it knows the highest truth and can judge it by its outer vision and mental opinions.

Approaches to Understand and Apply the Teachings

There are several approaches that we can recommend for studying and applying these teachings depending upon the level of insight and interest of the prospective aspirant. Note that all of these require that we study, meditate on, inquire, and apply these teachings in waking, dream, and deep sleep and in our interaction with society and the world of nature. Self-inquiry must become the very movement of our mind moment-to-moment, though beginning in certain phases, rhythms, and alignments with our life experience through body, prana, senses, and mind.

Examining the Teaching Systematically

Examine these teachings step by step through studying the text and noting the different stages of its teachings. Familiarize yourself with the different levels of its teachings, seeking to understand their progression, and how you can move through them in a systematic matter, practicing all the main factors involved in your own awareness and daily life.

Make sure that you deeply understand the core teachings of each verse, its implications, and practices before going on to the next verse. This requires carefully studying and deeply meditating upon each verse one by one and its relevance in our life and awareness. Be receptive to the teaching of each verse with a silent mind and let it reverberate within you. Don't try to judge it quickly by the opinions or speculations of our mind but contemplate its meaning in silence and receptivity.

You may need to stop after verses that deeply move you and take additional time to apply them, which may be for days, weeks or months before continuing to the next verse. Studying such a guidebook on Self-knowledge is not a question of simply reading a book or memorizing the key points involved as in a school program, hoping to pass a test, but of progressively turning one's awareness within and changing our perception of Self, world, and reality in a fundamental manner back into the Infinite. A radical change of awareness is the goal and proof of this inner learning, not any intellectual proficiency.

Examining the Teachings Most Relevant to Your Own Inner Search

Another helpful approach is to examine the portions of the text that appear most relevant to your current state of mind, situation in life, and level of inner development. Meditate upon these key insights until you have understood their essence, and integrated them into your daily life regimen, ultimately into your every moment awareness. You may need to spend much time on the preliminary teachings of the first verses, for example, which can be months or years, before moving on to the verse that are more advanced. You need to first develop a good foundation to hold your power of meditation to be able to understand the deeper teachings.

For example, you may first need to focus on control and calming of the prana and senses before trying to directly turn the mind within. The first section of the text may require extensive time and practice to master, preparing the ground for Self-inquiry later. See how ready you are for the deeper teachings by how you handle the difficulties of life and its conflicting dualities.

Holding to a Single Verse

Another approach is to choose one verse to focus on for a period of time to examine repeatedly, whether a day, a week or month. Truly understanding even a single verse will be highly transformative. This means trying to absorb the essence of the verse with our fullest attention and focusing on it as continually as possible in the movement of the mind.

You can focus on any particular verse that inspires you and try to open up to the depths of its meaning. You can see if any particular verse stands out and draws your attention. A certain teaching may be easier for us to understand or become motivated by than another, depending on our turn of thought, particular mindset, individual way of looking at reality or our stage and situation in life.

You can hold to a single verse until it permeates your awareness, like the main thought in your mind, whether it is hours or days. Then you can search for another specific verse to inspire you and go with the flow, rather than going through the text in only a sequential manner. Yet note that it is enough to gain the understanding of one verse to set our deeper Self-inquiry in motion, which we can then bring into the whole or our lives.

Examining the Teachings as the Voice of Your Inmost Self

Another approach is to examine the teachings according to your own Self-awareness, as if it arose spontaneously from inside you, a message from your own inner Being, not as a mere book or text or words of another but your own Self-revelation. Use the text like a mirror to look more deeply at your own Self and how your mind and consciousness works. Let the teaching and teacher merge into your own inner being in the spiritual heart (hridaya). Give up all sense of otherness in its examination, taking it as a special message to you from your inner eternal Being.

Learning the Sanskrit of the Text

We should note that learning the original Sanskrit of the text and its many levels of meaning, notably chanting the Sanskrit verses, can be very helpful, letting the resonance of the sounds vibrate within you according to their meaning and power in your own Consciousness. Sanskrit words have their own cadence and deeper meanings which are often untranslatable. Each verse is in the same special Sanskrit meter which has its own vibratory rhythm. Let your thoughts and your entire life be a mantric chant of joyous Self-realization.

Upadesha Saram is a sadhana teaching meant to be put into practice at an individual level, not simply to be read or casually thought about, much less made into an academic form of comparative study or semantic examination. It does not aim to propagate any theory or point of view in terms of philosophy, logic, or terminology. Its foundation is our own experience of Being and Consciousness as the Self within. It takes us back to the supreme reality that reveals itself once we let go of the dualistic mind and all attachments to mere words or ideas, speculations, or imaginations.

The Fire of Self Inquiry

This profound teaching is not just telling us that we are already Self-realized as we currently are in our ordinary lives and behavior, relative to our existing state of mind and personal desires. It directs us to the fiery tapas of Jnana Sadhana, to make that higher knowledge real within us. We must awaken that inner fire of Self-inquiry that burns away all other thoughts, tendencies, and karmas. We must learn to abide in that inner flame of awareness which shines eternally within us, let it consume us and unfold the deepest light within us, as a new birth in Self-awareness.

Meditation on Bhagavan Ramana Maharshi's Presence

Meditating upon Bhagavan Ramana's presence within oneself can be a great aid in this process of Self-inquiry. You can use his picture for this process as an additional aid. This should be done not simply to recognize Bhagavan at a personal level but to connect to the inner peace and Self-awareness that he radiated for all, and which continues to be accessible for serious aspirants.

For this purpose, the following Ramana mantra can be of benefit, which I have provided below along with a translation.

OM Namo Bhagavate Sri Ramaṇāya!
Arunācala Śivāya Namaḥ!

OM reverence to the
Bhagavan Sri Ramana!
To Shiva as the Arunachala Mountain
we surrender our hearts!

This mantra is to Bhagavan Ramana Maharshi as connected to Shiva of the sacred Arunachala Mountain where he resided in Tiruvannamalai and with which Ramana is identified. Arunachala is said to be the fire Linga of Shiva among the five element Lingas to Shiva in Tamil Nadu.

The mantra is used to call upon Ramana as Shiva and the mountain as reflecting our true Self and as the Universal Self. Shiva is said to be the Lord of the mountains. It reflects also Ramana's connection with the deity Skanda, son of Shiva and Uma, aid to be born of fire. The mountain is also said to be a Sri Yantra and to hold many Siddhas and great Yogis at a subtle level.

The Arunachaleshwar temple is one of the largest, most sacred, and honored in India where Ramana stayed and did his tapas as a youth. A special sacred fire is lit at the top of the mountain during the full Moon of the month of Kartika when the moon is in Krittika, Skanda as Kartikeya's Nakshatra, which is the Pleiades in western astronomy. This lighting of the fire is one of the main Hindu celebrations in South India. In other words, there is a great symbolism behind the mountain which has a long history in yogic teachings.

One may say, why should we use such mantras that we may not understand, which are merely words, sounds and ideas, and instead focus on the direct realization of our own Self apart from such extraneous considerations? Mantra aids in purifying the mind and unifying our mental focus as we have already discussed. It has an important role in all branches of Yoga, including, knowledge and devotion as indicated here.

Why should we invoke a person to guide us from within? some may also state, even a great guru like Ramana. The guru has a presence not merely as a person but as the guiding cosmic intelligence that we can connect to within. This guru can function as our inner guide if we are receptive to his grace and insight. Yet to contact such an inner guiding intelligence, we must have true devotion and inwardly surrender to the teacher, in recognition of the Self-knowledge he has embodied. Such *guru mantras* are most important for this purpose and form a whole type of yogic mantras along with deity mantras. In this chant both guru as Ramana and deity as Shiva are invoked.

By only our own personal efforts rooted in the body and ego mind, which are products of intractable ignorance, we cannot go far on the path of Self-Realization. We require an inner guidance to propel us forward, a connection with a teacher who has realized that supreme truth. It also helps to connect to a tradition or lineage holding that knowledge which we can align our minds and hearts with. Bhagavan Ramana can guide us in this process, whether we look to him directly or to teachers in his tradition to help us in our sadhana, extending to all ancient or modern masters of Advaita Vedanta.

The Maharshi teaches that you as a human being can realize the Self of the universe, which requires dissolving the mind and an inner death of the ego, which is very difficult to achieve or even approach. It cannot be imparted to us if we have not been purified of rajas and tamas, the qualities of agitation and inertia that prevail in the ordinary human being, and have developed a sattvic, dharmic and contemplative way of life. Mantra is the best way to purify the mind and make it sattvic. This Ramana mantra is the best way to contact his guidance and that of the Supreme Shiva, but it must be chanted with devotion, surrender and Self-inquiry.

May we have the humility, grace, and perseverance to approach that supreme Self-knowledge with utmost dedication, making the search for it the primary concern of our attention from waking to dream and deep sleep. When one is able to shut the mind off and merge into the inner consciousness at will, when there is a deep and unshakeable inner peace, when the thought of one's personal self in not there, then one is truly progressing along the way of Self-realization.

Then there is ultimately neither a path nor one who treads it; only a boundless light of awareness in all directions and into all dimensions within and without, ever unfolding itself, including and transcending the entire universe, the state of the Supreme Brahman.

May that Divine life of the bliss of the Self arise in all! We have the capacity to abide in that supreme *Atmananda,* but to dwell in that we must follow great gurus like Ramana and their teachings like *Upadesha Saram.*

Let us not forget our true Self that is the Self of all residing everywhere and upholding all of nature with our own true nature!

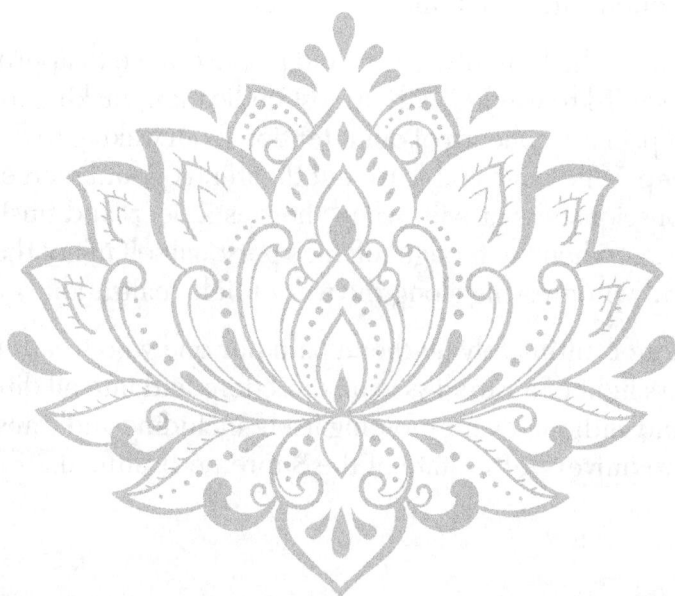

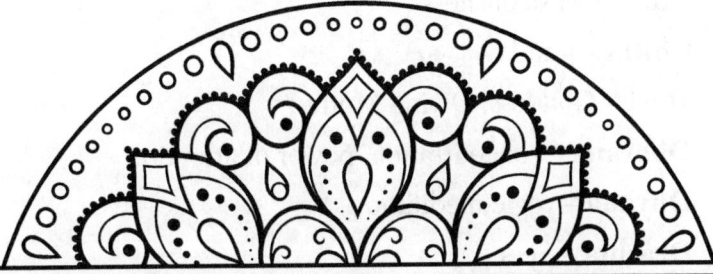

APPENDICES

Sanskrit Glossary

Acharya – Traditional teacher

Adhikara – Competence, capacity

Advaita – Non-duality

Agni – Fire as a cosmic principle of Self-awareness

Ahamkara – Ego or identification with body and mind

Ananda – Bliss, highest peace, contentment beyond thought

Atman – inner Self beyond body and mind

Atmavidya – Self-knowledge

Atma-Vichara – Self-inquiry as inquiry into the inner Self beyond the ego

Bhakti Yoga – Yoga of Devotion and Surrender

Bhagavan – Deity or Guru honored as one with the supreme Ananda

Brahman – Absolute, Supreme Reality of Being, Consciousness and Bliss

Brahma – Creative Power of Ishvara

Brahmavidya – Knowledge of Brahman

Buddhi – Discriminating intelligence

Chit – Consciousness

Chitta – mind

Devi – Goddess, Divine Mother

Dharana – concentration, power of attention

Dhyana – yogic meditation

Drashta – Seer

Ekagra chitta – one-pointed mind

Ganesha/Ganapati – cosmic intelligence, son of Shiva, symbolized by an elephant

Hatha Yoga – Yoga of Prana and psycho-physical techniques

Ishvara – Ruling Consciousness behind the universe, Creator, Preserver and Dissolver of all

Jivatman – Individual Atman or Self in the process of Karma and Rebirth

Jnana Yoga – Yoga of Self-knowledge

Karma Yoga – Yoga of Service and right action

Mahat – Cosmic intelligence

Manas – mind

Moksha – liberation of Consciousness

OM – Sound of the Self, cosmic sound vibration

Paramananda – Supreme Bliss

Paramatman – Supreme Self beyond all manifestation

Prakriti – manifest world of nature

Puja – Devotional forms of ritual and worship

Purusha – Self, Person, Atman

Raja Yoga – Yoga of calming and controlling the mind, turning the awareness within

Rajas (three gunas) – quality of aggression and ego.

Sadhaka –Aspirant engaged in a path of Self-realization

Sadhana – Yoga practice in various yogic disciplines

Sakshi bhava – state of the witnessing observer

Sat – Being, Sadvidya as Knowledge of Being

Shankara, Shankaracharya – Great teacher of Advaita Vedanta

Shakti – Goddess as the Cosmic Power

Shiva – Supreme Consciousness, Transcendent power of Ishvara

Skanda, Murugan – Son of Shiva and Parvati connected to Agni

Sushupti – State of deep sleep, in which mind and body consciousness is withdrawn

Tamas (three gunas) – quality of ignorance and darkness

Tapas – Yogic self-discipline and purificatory practices

Vairagya – Detachment

Vedanta – Vedic knowledge system rooted in Upanishads, Bhagavad Gita and Brahma

Sutras, as well as special Vedantic texts

Vedas – Mantras of the ancient Rishis from the early ancient period setting forth the teachings of Yoga, Vedanta and Vedic Sciences

Vichara – Inquiry, as Self-Inquiry, Atma Vichara

Vishnu – Sustaining power of Ishvara

Viveka – Inner discernment

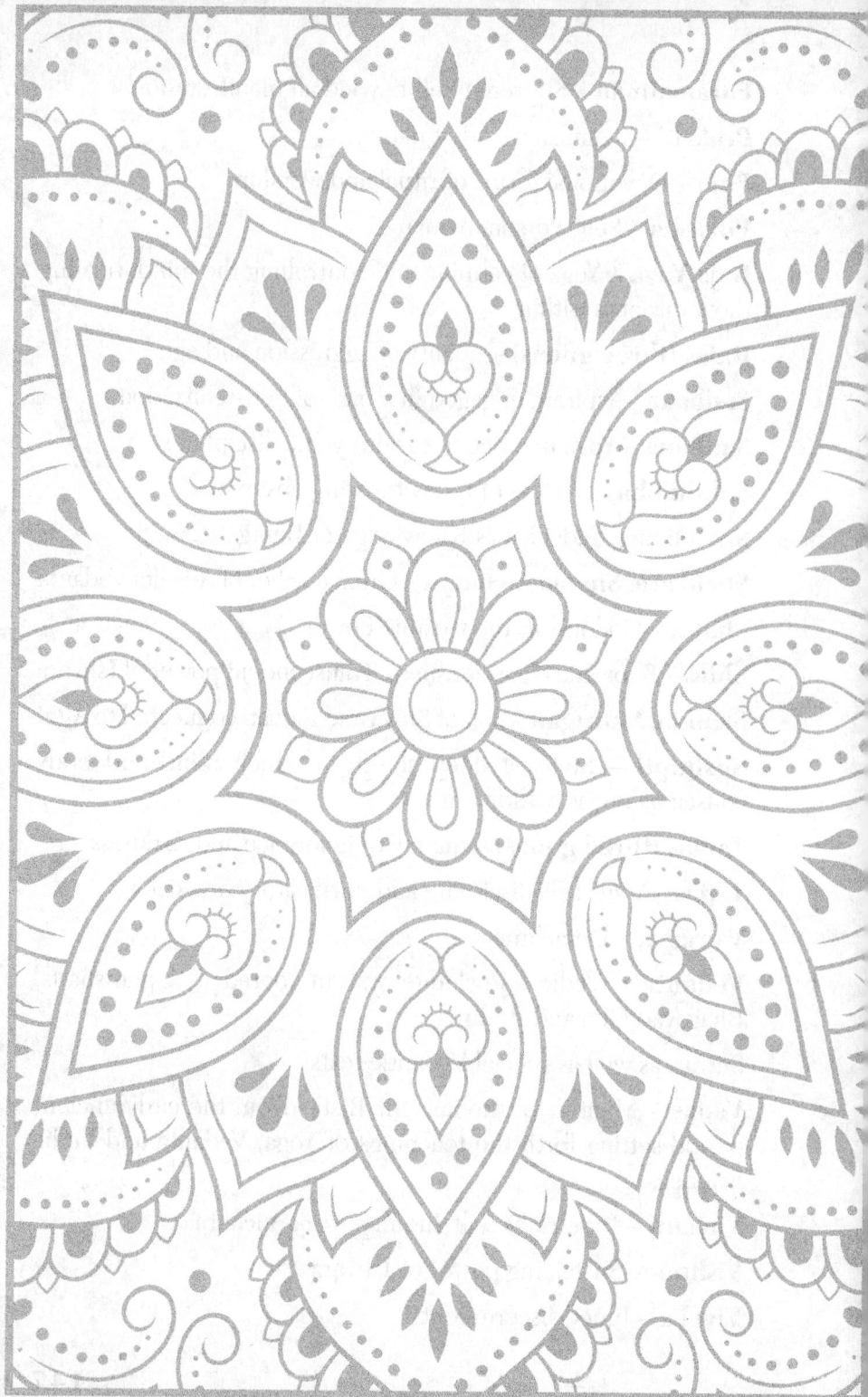

NOTE ON THE AUTHOR

Dr. David Frawley D.Litt. (Pandit Vamadeva Shastri b.1950) is Vedacharya, an internationally recognized Vedacharya (Vedic teacher), adept in the fields of Yoga, Vedanta, Ayurveda, and Vedic astrology. He has shared this Vedic wisdom through programs, books, and publications over the past forty years, extending to more than fifty books in twenty languages worldwide. He has been one of the main western born gurus to bring these Vedic sciences to the world.

Dr. Frawley is the director of the American Institute of Vedic Studies (www.vedanet.com) an online center sharing his teachings, which offers online courses, articles, programs, retreats, and webinars, along with his wife Yogini Shambhavi.

Vamadeva is a rare recipient of the prestigious Padma Bhushan (2015), the third highest civilian award of the government of India for his work in Vedic education. He received a National Eminence Award from the South India Education Society (SIES) in Mumbai, India. He has D.Litt. degrees (doctor of letters) from SVYASA University (Swami Vivekananda Yoga Anusandhana Samsthana) in Bangalore and another D.Litt. from Ram Manohar Lohia University in Ayodhya, Uttar Pradesh. He has helped found Ayurvedic and Vedic Astrology schools and associations in many countries.

Vamadeva is a prominent voice representing Hinduism/ Sanatana Dharma and is connected to many ashrams and organizations including the Sri Ramanashram, Sri Aurobindo

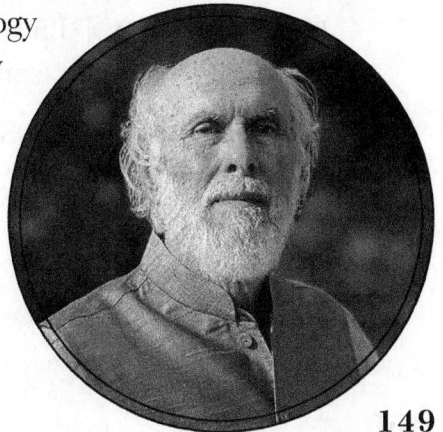

Ashram, BAPS Swaminarayan, Chinmaya Mission, Swami Dayananda Arsha Vidya, Vivekananda Kendra and many more. He has done programs with with the Indian Council of Cultural Relations (ICCR), Indian Council of Historical Research (IHCR), and the Ministry of AYUSH. His work is well known and has been followed in India over the last thirty years.

He has been an Advisor for the National Consortium of Ayurvedic Professionals, Hindu American Foundation (HAF) and for the City of Auroville in India.

Vamadeva has followed the teachings of Bhagavan Ramana Maharshi and Ganapati Muni for many years and has discussed them in depth in his various books like *Vedic Yoga: the Path of the Rishi, Shiva the Lord of Yoga, Vedantic Meditation, Mantra Yoga and Primal Sound, Inner Tantric Yoga* and *Tantric Yoga and the Wisdom Goddesses.*

Dr. Frawley has several social media accounts, writes extensively for various India publications, and has made many appearances on the India media.

www.vedanet.com

@drdavidfrawley | Facebook

@davidfrawleyved | X (formerly Twitter)

@drdavidfrawley | Linked In
https://www.linkedin.com/in/david-frawley-275a98266/

American Institute of Vedic Studies Information

www.vedanet.com

The Works of David Frawley

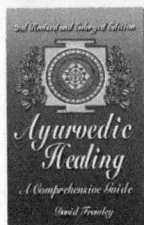

Ayurvedic Healing
A Comprehensive Guide, 2nd Revised and Enlarged Edition
David Frawley • 468 pp pb • $24.95 • ISBN: 978-0-9149-5597-9

Ayurvedic Healing presents Ayurvedic treatments for over eighty common diseases and ailments, from the common cold to cancer. This extraordinary manual of ayurvedic health care offers the ancient system of mind-body medicine to the modern reader. Treatment methods include traditional approaches using diet, herbs, oils, gems, mantra and meditation for today's health concerns. Learn empowering Ayurvedic lifestyle practices and daily health considerations for your personal mind-body type! Revised and expanded edition.

Ayurveda, Nature's Medicine
David Frawley & Dr. Subhash Ranade
368 pp pb • $19.95 • ISBN: 978-0-9149-5595-5

Ayurveda, Nature's Medicine details India's extraordinary natural healing traditions rooted in five thousand years of practice. The Ayurvedic "science of life" is a mind-body system that includes physical, psychological and spiritual healing. This book explains Ayurvedic approaches to all levels of wellness, including diagnostic and treatment methods, and the healing techniques of diet, herbs, yoga and meditation. It shares the wisdom of daily and seasonal regimes for optional health and vitality, along with lifestyle recommendations concerning exercise, sexuality and diet.

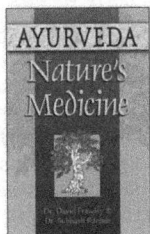

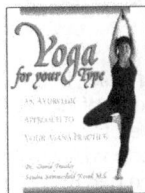

Yoga for Your Type
David Frawley & Sandra Summerfield, M.S.
296 pp • $29.95 • ISBN: 978-0-9102-6130-2

Discover the Yoga asanas (Yoga poses) best suited to your individual type according to Ayurvedic wisdom! Yoga and Ayurveda have been long regarded as effective methods for holistic care and chronic pain management. Balance your energy and restore well-being with healing systems based on 5,000 years of practice! Yoga for Your Type integrates the foundations of these systems and presents a customized approach for your personal wellness.

Yoga and Ayurveda
Self-Healing and Self-Realization
David Frawley • 360 pp pb • $19.95 • ISBN: 978-0-9149-5581-8

Applied together, Yoga and Ayurveda open pathways to optimal health, vitality and higher awareness. Yoga and Ayurveda reveals the secrets hidden in our body, breath, senses, mind and chakras, and provides transformational methods to unlock these inner powers. Learn how diet, herbs, asana, pranayama and meditation hold the key to whole-being improvement and life-changing growth. The first book of its kind published in the West, Yoga and Ayurveda remains a must-read for anyone exploring these topics.

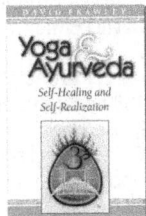

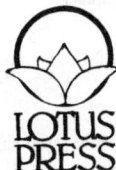

The Works of David Frawley

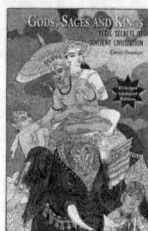

Gods, Sages and Kings
Vedic Secrets of Ancient Civilization, Revised and Enlarged
David Frawley • 416 pp • $22.95 • ISBN: 978-0-9102-6137-1

Gods, Sages and Kings presents a remarkable accumulation of evidence pointing to the existence of a common spiritual culture in the ancient world from which present civilization may be more of a decline than an advance. The book is based upon new interpretation of the ancient Vedic teachings of India, and brings out many new insights from this unique source often neglected and misinterpreted in the West. In addition, it discusses recent archaeological discoveries in India whose implications are now only beginning to emerge.

Inner Tantric Yoga
Frawley, David • 280 pp • $19.95 • ISBN: 978-0-9406-7650-3

Inner Tantric Yoga presents the deeper tradition of Tantra, its multidimensional vision of the Divine and its transformative practices of mantra and meditation that take us far beyond the outer models of how Tantra is usually presented today. The book can expand your horizons about masculine and feminine energies, Self and world, universe and the Absolute into a living experience of the Infinite and Eternal both within and around you.

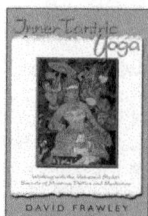

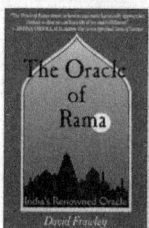

The Oracle of Rama
India's Renowned Oracle
David Frawley • 204 pp • $12.95 • ISBN: 978-0-9102-6135-7

The Oracle of Rama shows us how we can make karmically appropriate choices so that we can live a life of joy and fulfillment states Deepak Chopra. The Oracle Of Rama is perhaps the greatest oracle of India, as well as one of the simplest and easiest to use. The Oracle of Rama uses the insights of Tulsidas, one of the greatest seers of the Vedic traditions, to unlock the secrets of the realm of unmanifest intelligence and open up for us all the creative potentials of the universe. - Deepak Chopra

The Yoga of Herbs
Ayurvedic Guide to Herbal Medicine, 2nd Revised and Enlarged Edition
David Frawley & Dr. Vasant Lad • 288 pp • $19.95 • ISBN: 978-0-9415-2424-7

For the first time, here is a detailed explanation and classification of herbs, using the ancient system of Ayurveda. More than 270 herbs are listed, with 108 herbs explained in detail. Included are many of the most commonly used western herbs with a profound Ayurvedic perspective. Important Chinese and special Ayurvedic herbs are introduced. Beautiful diagrams and charts, as well as detailed glossaries, appendices and index are included.

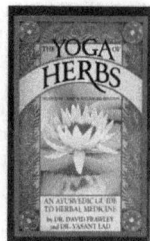

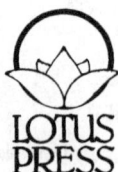